VEGAN WITH NOUR

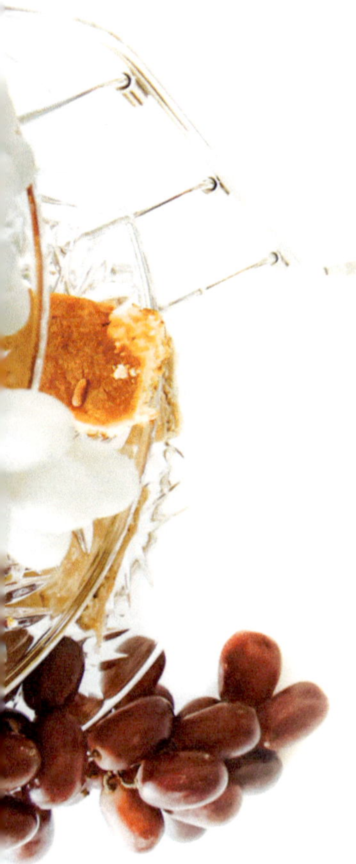

VEGAN WITH NOUR

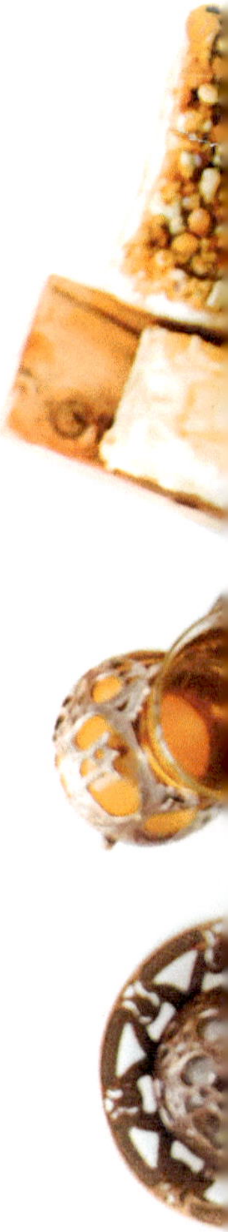

NOUR DANNO

FOREWORD BY
JOHN SALLEY

Publisher: Nour Danno
Michigan, USA.
248-840-6354
www.VeganWithNour.com

Ordering Information:
Quantity sales. Special discounts are available on quantity purchases by corporations, associations, and others. For details contact the publisher: 248-840-6354 or visit www.VeganWithNour.com

Danno, Nour.
Vegan with Nour.
p. cm.
Cover Photography: Alyssa Leffler Photography, for Snap + Social + Solve
Styling: Christina Brillati, Tribe Detroit
Editor: Geoffrey Sperl, The Wordsmithing Studio, www.TheWordsmithing.Studio
Book Design: Quileen Adams, for Creative Hina Design LLC, www.CreativeHina.com
Main Food Photography: Quileen Adams, for Creative Hina Design LLC
Animal Photography: Mago photography

ISBN 978-1-7347619-0-0
1. Nutrition 2. Cooking 3. Health

To Teta Amena

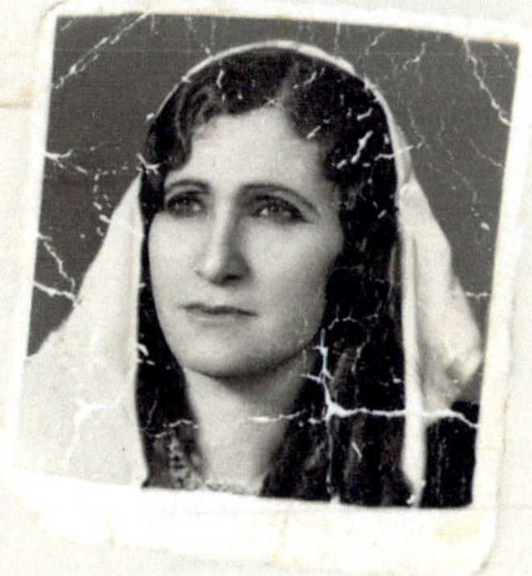

I dedicate this book to Teta Amena, who was not only my beloved grandmother, but my favorite person in world.

Teta worked hard to raise her kids after her husband died when she was only 27. She became a cook in order to provide for their eight children. She became so good, she came to cook at Socrate, a famous restaurant on Hamra Street in Beirut. She worked there for over 30 years, with my aunt taking care of my mother and her siblings when they were young.

She was the one who taught me how to cook. I grew up watching teta taking care of us all, cooking the healthiest food ever. Her kitchen was very special, simple and clean. The only oil she used was olive oil. She had very big jars of red and yellow lentils, chickpeas, and burghul. She used to hang all her pots and utensils in front of her and within reach. I remember her hanging okra on a chain right next to her little cute old fridge (which I would open five times or more every time I visited). From Lebanese mujaddara to Turkish kibbeh, my teta was, in my eyes, the best cook in world.

Her passing in November 2016 broke my heart. Teta Amena taught me to be grateful and how to work hard, be loving, be respectful, and be good. She was—and still is—the ideal I try to live up to.

CONTENTS

FOREWORD

The first time I met Nour, I knew she was going to be a vegan star.

She has all the qualities—enthusiastic, attractive, smart, and always speaking out for animal rights. We need more people like her.

Many of us grew up eating meat or wearing leather, but today that's different—we've all learned how great a vegan lifestyle is! We just don't need animals' flesh, blood, or skin to survive like we did so many years ago.

Animals have rights—just like humans. It's prejudice that lets us deny rights—ones we expect ourselves—to others. Regardless of what that discrimination is based on—gender, race, or species—it is not acceptable. Consider pigs and dogs. We keep dogs as pets and beloved family companions, but we eat pigs. They both have a similar capacity to feel pain, are similarly intelligent, and emotionally complex animals. But we allow prejudice based on species to tell us one is a companion and the other is food.

Go vegan. *Vegan with Nour* will help you make the transition. Eat plenty of vegetables and fruit, legumes, and nuts, and drink water with nutrients. I love her recipes and natural remedies. She also highlights the health and medicinal benefits of herbs and spices, of which I am a big believer in. You won't have an excuse not to go vegan after reading *Vegan with Nour*.

Give it a try and enjoy it! ☺

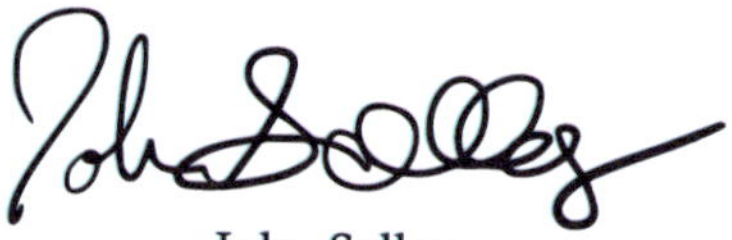

John Salley,
Four-time NBA champion and first
player to win with three franchises

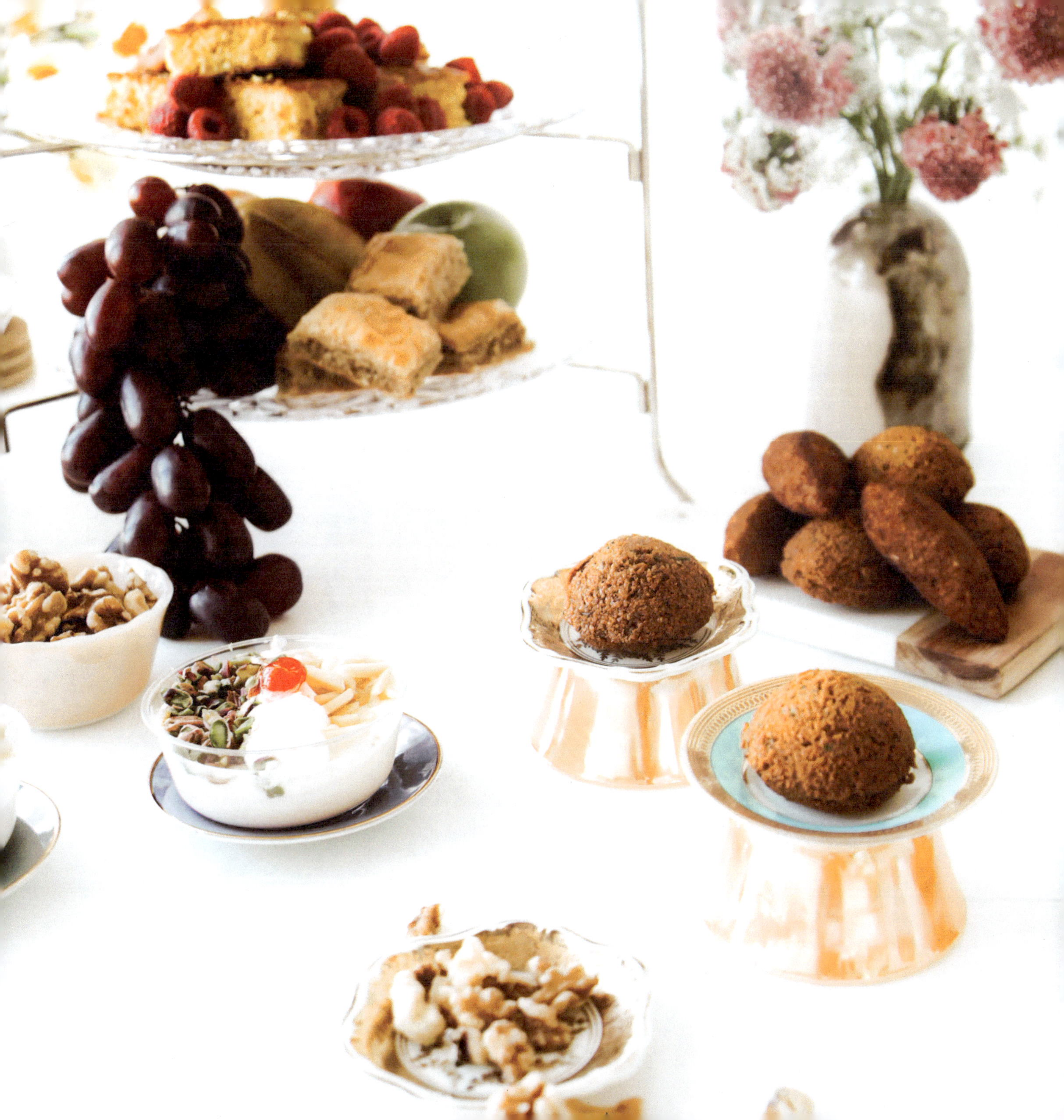

INTRODUCTION

GROWING UP

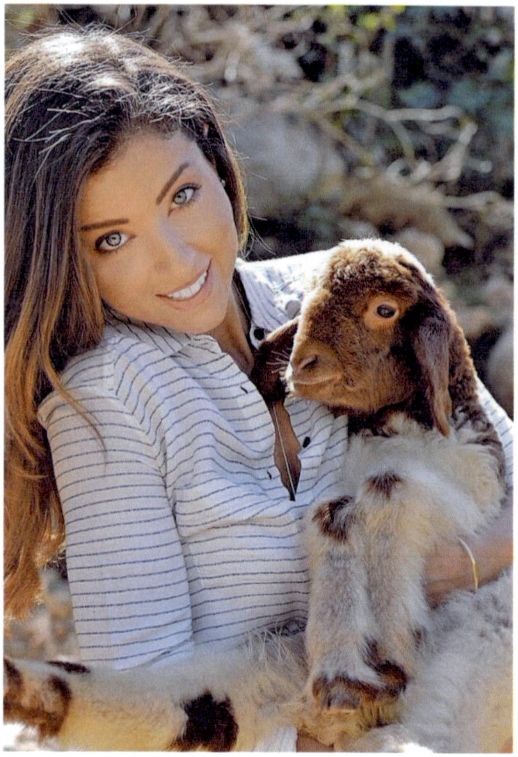

"You should be a nutritionist." It's what they all used to tell me when I was a kid in Lebanon. While all the other kids were enjoying their potato chips and chocolate bars, I was busy reading the nutrition facts. My mother tells me that, even as a child, I was always obsessed with eating healthy. I guess it was no surprise I decided to study nutrition and fitness at Notre Dame University in Lebanon or that I've become vegan. There's a little voice inside me, pushing me forward, and that's the reason I've always believed I have something to say about nutrition and fitness to the world.

I was born in January of 1992 (my mother tells me it was one of the coldest nights in Lebanon's history) to a modest family—my father is a hairdresser and my mother is a housewife—and we lived in a congested Beruit neighborhood, where the houses are very close to one another. My mother used to send plates of food to our neighbor, and they would do the same. She can make all different kinds of Lebanese and Mediterranean dishes—kibbeh, tabbouleh, hummus, loubya b'ziet, baba ghanoush, mulukhiyah, couscous, yabrak... you name it, she makes it. She's a great cook—and she learned that from her mother.

I remember my grandmother's hands. I learned to cook from her—including tips that she discovered on her own and used for herself (like mixing pomegranate molasses with lemon, sumac, olive oil, and salt as a dressing for tabbouleh and fattoush, and how to use chickpeas)—but it's her hands, and how she used to make the kibbeh with her pinky finger, that I remember vividly (not that I eat traditional kibbeh).

I come from a Muslim family, and yes, Muslims do eat beef, lamb, chicken, and fish. I do not. Even as a child, I was always against hurting animals, and I have been vegetarian for a long time (and went vegan in 2015) because of that. When it comes to Islam and food, there are some unique rules they believe in—eating pork is forbidden, for example, because of its cloven hoof and the fact it eats other animals. There are also strong scientific reasons not to eat them (as pork can be a carrier for parasites and bacteria), as well as ethical reasons (pigs for slaughter are typically kept in small crates, surrounded by their feces). Having been raised in a religion and culture that already forbids specific foods may have helped me in my journey.

My family supports me (even if it's counter to their beliefs), though I suppose they thought I was always different, always wanting to prove a point to them (and everyone else). For example, I convinced my cousin to stop hunting because it is barbaric and morally wrong. And, when I was 10, I rescued my uncle's goat from being slaughtered. He was preparing for Eid meal and was going to grill the meat. I didn't allow them to kill it. I began sobbing, and I still remember the look this goat had—it was terrified, and I promise it was crying. I simply could not understand why this

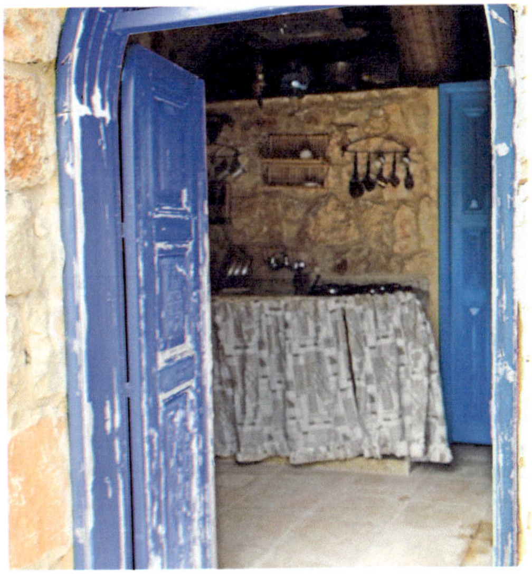

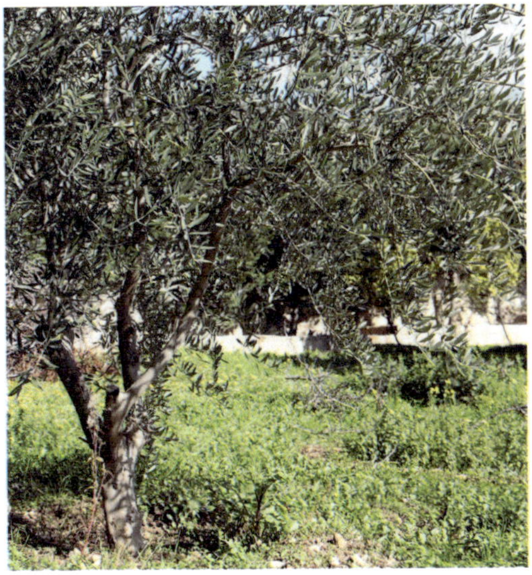

animal had to die. I managed to keep him from slaughtering the goat—even he felt sorry for it by the time I was done standing my ground. Since that time, my family has understood and supported my vegetarian and veganism.

NOW

My husband also supports me and I cook vegan meals at home almost every day (thought we might order from the very few local vegan restaurants near our home in Michigan). Many of those around me support me and believe in veganism, especially after I opened their eyes as to why we shouldn't eat eggs or meat.

In this book, I use the terms "vegan" and "plant-based" in different ways. It's important to understand I see veganism as a lifestyle, not just a diet. We shouldn't eat, wear, or use any animal products, and we should be respectful of their lives as independent beings. That's what I see as veganism and what I mean when I write "vegan." When referring specifically to food, I may write "plant-based," but please understand I am firm in my belief that is only one part of the overall vegan lifestyle. I believe once we are convinced to stop eating animals, then we will be against using animals in the circus, or wearing their fur, and so on. What I've realized is that some people are simply unaware. For example, I convinced my father to go vegan after showing him how animals are tortured at the slaughterhouses, and I convinced my very good friend to stop wearing fur after explaining to her how the skin is removed. This is a mission for me.

My life changed after adopting a vegan lifestyle, and my health improved—no more acne or constipation. Choosing a vegan diet also didn't hinder me from reaching my fitness goals, and it is giving me a nice boost of added energy and strength. But I feel I can go further than just me.

I didn't realize it until I came to America, but veganism is big now. You can usually find restaurants with vegan plates on the menu; on your social media feed, you read the word "vegan" on someone's post almost every time. While I have been vegan for a while, I rarely heard anything about it. After moving, I started to hear more and more about veganism in discussions—that simply doesn't happen in Lebanon. I feel somewhat less alone being a vegan in America.

WHY SHOULD WE GO VEGAN?

Perhaps you already are, so I hope I can add to what you know! If you're curious, then I hope I can make a strong argument for going vegan.

My reasons for going vegan are mixed. To start, which is clear from the story about the goat, I have always loved animals and believe they have their own lives—ones we shouldn't be controlling. I am also living with Hashimoto's thyroiditis[1] (better known as "Hashimoto's disease" or just "Hashimoto's"), and, because of that, I need to manage my diet and work against the weight gain it can cause. For those reasons, I was a vegetarian for most of my life. I stayed vegetarian until I watched the documentary *What the Health*[2] (which you can watch on their website) in 2017, and the arguments it made convinced me to go vegan.

Now, it's unlikely you have Hashimoto's, but there are plenty of health reasons for a woman to go vegan. A plant-based diet lowers your risk for various ailments, such as heart disease and Type 2 diabetes.[3] Because animal products do not contain any carbohydrates and are higher in fat, it's more challenging to stay fit—dietary fat has more calories and is more easily converted into body fat.[4] The calorie density of animal products can lead to us overeating them (while vegans can load up our plates with veggies and still be lean).[5] A plant-based diet, by removing the animal-based fat, also can lower your body mass index (BMI) significantly.

A plant based diet will help save you from heart disease, cholesterol, and various cancers

Furthermore, food from animals can get "dirty" easily. People for the Ethical Treatment of Animals (PETA) states on their website, "Every time you sit down to a meal containing meat, eggs, or dairy products, you're dining on known carcinogens, bacteria, and other contaminants that can accumulate in your body and remain there for years. Animal products are loaded with bacteria, antibiotics, hormones, dioxins, and a host of other toxins that can cause serious health problems in humans."[6]

Many people fear a loss of energy or muscle mass when abstaining from animal products, but quite the opposite is true—we can improve our fitness when we quit consuming animal products.[7]

Dairy may add to arthritis pain, and that's because of a protein they contain.[8] For some people, this protein can irritate and inflame the tissue around their joints. Not only that, it may cause severe disease, including a correlation between dairy fat intake and ovarian cysts and ovarian cancer,[9] and some who think the protein in milk can actually cause osteoporosis.[10] Furthermore, as you probably know from the move towards "organic" foods, many farmers in the dairy industry artificially introduce hormones to make their cows produce more. Studies have started to explore, amongst other things, whether those hormones can trigger acne (and, in observing my clients, I've seen a reduction in acne when dairy is cut).[11]

Besides, meat and dairy are hard to digest and use a lot of your energy, possibly leaving you tired.[12] A vegan diet doesn't stop you from reaching your fitness goals—and might boost your energy and strength. As you can see in my case, veganism can help your skin clear up and better your digestion. Removing fatty foods from a diet seems to reduce acne, and vegetables can make your skin healthier due to their minerals and vitamins. Further, their dietary fiber helps with digestion and elimination of toxins which, in turn, clears up your skin even more.[13][14]

In *How Not to Die*, Dr. Michael Greger tells us eating a plant-based diet, and just walking every day, can improve our bodies' defenses against cancer within a few weeks. Greger mentions researchers who ran tests of women before and just after 14 days of healthy living, introducing their blood to breast cancer cells. The blood taken after the women started eating healthier was shown to suppress cancer growth significantly better, with a marked decrease in cancer cell growth. The researchers attributed this effect to the reduced intake of animal protein.

If we won't hurt our pets, then why do we hurt cows or pigs or fish or chicken?

The second reason is ethical. If we won't hurt our pets, then why do we hurt cows or pigs or fish or chicken? Do you think cattle graze in a field, enjoying the warm green grass? Actually, they're confined in dirt feedlots without a blade of grass. Their tails are cut without any painkiller. Invasive, nonconsensual rectal, and vaginal penetration is used in artificial insemination. Dairy cows are injected with hormones to increase their yield, their calves are taken from them, and, often around four years of age, they're slaughtered as they can no longer produce

Chickens are always under stress, living their lives in small cages. The cages may be stacked on top of one another, allowing waste to fall onto birds in the lower cages. They often die in their cages, and dead chickens are sometimes left in the same spaces as those still living.

Pigs are actually complex animals and very intelligent.[15] Some people keep pigs as pets because of how complex they are. Could you imagine eating your dog? On factory farms, they're forced to live in their own waste and sometimes even amid the corpses of other pigs. They spend their lives in tiny crates where they're unable to turn or even lie down comfortably. And they, much like cows, are repeatedly impregnated until they are slaughtered.

Stop picking up dead animals at the store or eating them at restaurants! No innocent living creature should suffer from pain for our sake. Do you need more evidence to understand how animals are treated? How about that dairy cows are forcibly impregnated (through non-consensual artificial insemination) to keep them at peak lactation? The dairy farmers take the calf from her right after it's born so they can then take her milk, so if we feel for a human mother suffering because she lost her child, what about this cow? Aside from the cow's feelings, what about the pain the animals go through? We can stop it all with a plant-based diet.

The third reason is environmental. PETA points out raising livestock for consuming meat uses up resources (taking almost 2,400 gallons of water for a pound of cow flesh), pollute the air (due to dust and gasses emitted from farms), and pollute the water (with the farm run-off along the Mississippi River helping cause the dead zone in the Gulf of Mexico!).[16]

If you're not an animal or climate activist and you aren't interested in those causes, then do it for your health! As PETA points out, "Research has shown that vegetarians are 50 percent less likely to develop heart disease, and meat-eaters are nine times more likely to be obese than pure vegetarians are. 70 percent of [the animals] have pneumonia by the time they're sent to the slaughterhouse."[17] Dr. Joel Kahn—a top cardiologist, well-known vegan doctor, and a friend—thinks plant-based nutrition is the best preventative medicine. In his book The Plant-Based Solution, he states the "case for plant-based diets preventing and reversing heart disease is without a doubt the strongest compared to other diet claiming to modify chronic diseases worldwide"[18]

As you can see, I am passionate about this topic. I guess what the others used to tell me was somewhat right—I did end up graduating with a double major in nutrition and physical education. But instead of a nutritionist, I want to focus on helping women with their health and fitness by working with them to find a plant-based diet that sustains them and exercise that fulfills them. We simply eat animals for pleasure and out of tradition. If you ask your mother why she's using meat in her kitchen, she'd tell you about protein and nutrients animal products provide, that she's used to it, and she doesn't know how to make your favorite meal without using animal products.

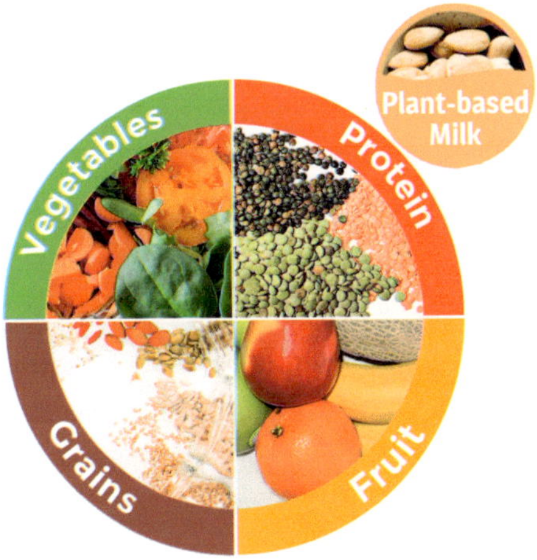

Who said protein only exists in meat products? Who said only cow's milk provides you with calcium? Your mother and your grandmother? The commercials on TV? The United States Department of Agriculture (USDA) has had some effect over the past century. If you're not familiar with the American "food pyramid," it's one of the best known of their food guides.[19] The idea of a guide was first introduced in 1916 in order to provide science-based dietary guidance to Americans. For years, the guides focused on animal products delivering your protein, fat, and various vitamins. Your grandparents and parents grew up with these in school and on TV—it's what they were told a balanced diet should look like.

The current version of the guide, MyPlate, pulls back on the animal products somewhat (just calling-out "protein," as opposed to "meat and poultry," but still keeps a label for "dairy"). I suggest making your own "plate" (like I have) and including vegetables, protein, grains, and fruits along with non-dairy sources of milk and cheese. Hopefully, the USDA will come up with something like our plates, because meat and dairy is killing us.

After studying nutrition and physical education, and researching it, I was convinced we don't need animals to get all the nutrients we need—we may even live longer without it. It's also beyond health for me—I cannot hurt animals. It's my ideology—I have my own beliefs that animals have feelings, so we can't kill them, and animals aren't our belongings, so we can't wear them or eat them.

Things have changed. We can explain to our parents that we can get protein, carbs, and fat from plants. There is no proof, whatsoever, that human beings must eat animal products to be healthy and thriving. When we go vegan, we tend to try new food and new dishes. Have you ever had a quinoa salad? How about black bean burgers? A Buddha bowl? When you think of the fact there are at least 20,000 species of edible plants, and, likely, you haven't tried a third of them yet!

I wrote this because a little voice inside my head is telling me to share with others (especially women) why we don't and shouldn't have to kill animals for food or clothes, how we can get plant sources of nutrients we need, and how being vegan, in conjunction with fitness, can help women live better lives. I have many of my grandmother's recipes, and I'll be sharing them (adapted to be vegan if necessary) through the book. Admittedly, my grandmother wasn't vegan and was of a different time, but she taught me how heavily plant-based the diets of older generations of Lebanese and Turks were. They barely ate meat or chicken, and fish wasn't an option—plants were vital to surviving there, and we can use a lot of her knowledge to create tasty, traditional dishes with a vegan spin. In addition to the recipes, I will go over my daily routine and discuss the ingredients I use and why.

Vegan Protein sources

10g Soy products *Such as tofu per ½ cup*	**2g Chia Seeds** *per tablespoon*
15 g Tempeh *per ½ cup*	**5g Hemp Seeds** *per tablespoon*
9.2 g Edamame *per ½ cup*	**8g Potatoes** *per serving*
8.84 g Lentils *per ½ cup*	**4g Broccoli** *medium stalk*
7.25 g Chickpeas *per ½ cup*	**2g Kale** *per cup*
20.5g Peanuts *per ½ cup*	**8g Cooked Quinoa** *per cup*
16.5g Almonds *per ½ cup*	**3g Mushrooms** *Five Medium*

Starting the transition to a plant-based diet and a vegan lifestyle can be easy. For example:

Eat a rainbow of fruits and vegetables to start. Find out what you like!

» I'm biased toward chickpeas because, when it comes to the cornerstones of the Lebanese kitchen, chickpeas are even more critical than salt. And what was utterly unknown to the early people in the Middle East was how good for you they are! They lower levels of LDL cholesterol, provide omega-3 fatty acids, manganese, folate, copper, dietary fiber, phosphorus, protein, iron, and zinc in addition to many other benefits. Plus, they taste yummy!

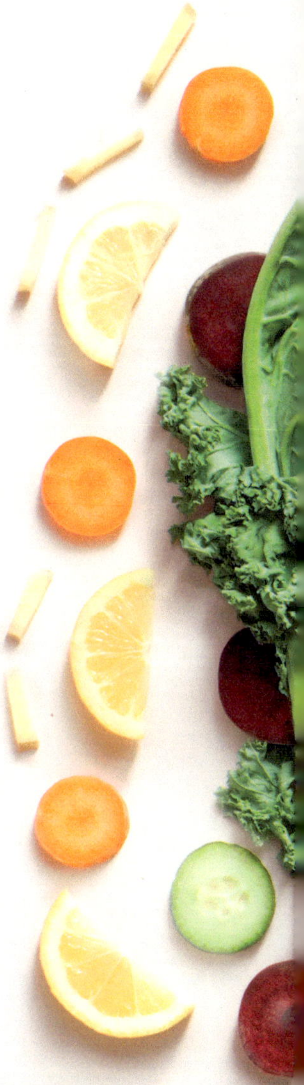

Eat higher fiber starchy foods—oats, sweet potatoes, whole wheat bread and pasta, and always choose brown rice over white!

Include reliable sources of protein:

» soy is the most commonly talked about, with tofu (and other similar soy products) having 10 g, tempeh having 15 g, and edamame having 9.2 g (all per ½ cup);

» then legumes and nuts, such as lentils with 8.84 g, chickpeas with 7.25 g, almonds (16.5 g), and peanuts with a whopping 20.5 g (again, these are all per ½ cup);

» seeds, such as quinoa (8 g per cooked cup), chia (2 g per tablespoon, or over 27 g per cup), and hemp (5 g per tablespoon, or over 65 g per cup);

» some more traditional vegetables, like broccoli (4 g per medium stalk), kale (2 g per cup), mushrooms (3 g per five medium ones), and potatoes (8 g per cup)

» and, if you dislike or can't eat of those due to a sensitivity or an allergy, there are supplements like spirulina, which delivers 8 g of protein per 2 tablespoons.

Be sure to eat foods with the vitamins and minerals (either naturally occurring or fortified) you need:

» it's vital for women to eat calcium-rich foods daily, such as green beans, soybean sprouts, okra, broccoli, or something like calcium-set tofu;

» make sure you have a reliable source of iodine like kombu kelp and wakame;

» you need to make sure you are getting enough zinc to help boost your immune system, so hemp seeds, oatmeal, tofu, squash seeds can help with that;

» we all need our iron, and a lot of amazing foods are rich in it—lentils, soybeans, tofu, tempeh,

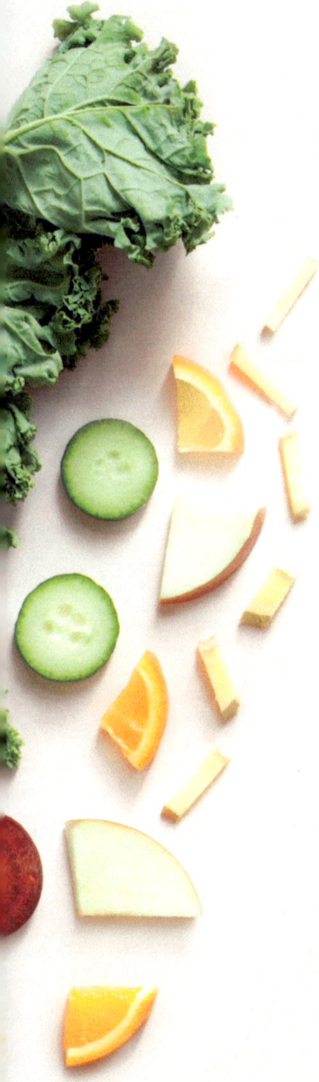

lima beans, black beans, chickpeas, quinoa, brown rice, pumpkin, squash, pine, pistachio, sunflower, and cashews (to name only a few); to help absorbing iron, make sure to eat plenty of fruit with high amounts of vitamin C, like oranges, plums, or chili peppers (you could also eat food rich in both iron and vitamin C, like broccoli and bok choy);

» get enough vitamin D, either through fortified non-dairy milk, fortified tofu, cremini mushrooms (that have been exposed to ultraviolet light), or a supplement (you can get some from exposure to the sun, too, but be careful!);

» and very importantly, when it comes to red blood cell production and growth and development in children, make sure you get enough vitamin B12 Unfortunately, that is mostly synthesized through meat and eggs, so the best way to get it is through a B12 supplement (and through fortified cereals or yeast).

You still need fats, so use oil high in unsaturated fats, such as olive oil, and use nuts and seeds, rich in omega-3 fatty acids—walnuts, chia, and flaxseed.
And in terms of your health:

» use herbs and spices, not salt, when you season your food (it may take a little while to get used to not using salt everywhere, but it's worth it);

» drink six to eight glasses of water each day (this is dependent on your weight and height, so find a calculator online to help guide you);

» keep active—even if you just walk a few miles a day!

Remember, you are the choices that you make, so make the right ones. Be active, healthy, and positive. It's all connected one to another—the toxins we find in meat affect our lives in many ways. If you keep the idea in mind that our actions in each area of our lives affect the other activities, you will begin to feel the change. As you change, you will help make a change globally. Starting in your own home and switching to a vegan lifestyle will not only improve your health, but it will help the entire world. Eating animals enables an industry that affects the environment—in the air and water and other ways—as they process the billions and billions of animals raised for meat, eggs, and milk in America each year.[20]

I'm not saying my way is the only way to do this, but it's worked for me and others in my life, so I think it may work for you, too. So, thank you for being interested and for going on this journey with me! Let's begin, shall we?

ENDNOTES

1. https://en.wikipedia.org/wiki/Hashimoto's_thyroiditis
2. https://www.whatthehealthfilm.com/
3. https://www.health.harvard.edu/staying-healthy/the-right-plant-based-diet-for-you
4. https://nutriciously.com/high-carb-low-fat-vegan-diet/
5. https://www.huffpost.com/entry/meat-hunger-is-real-for-some-people-not-you_b_9632646
6. https://www.peta.org/living/food/meat-contamination/
7. https://www.medicalnewstoday.com/articles/321477.php
8. https://www.pcrm.org/health-topics/arthritis
9. https://www.ncbi.nlm.nih.gov/pmc/articles/PMC4876783/
10. https://nutritionfacts.org/2017/01/31/why-is-milk-consumption-associated-with-more-bone-fractures/
11. https://www.pcrm.org/news/health-nutrition/dairy-linked-acne-development
12. https://www.onegreenplanet.org/natural-health/signs-your-body-doesnt-dig-dairy/
13. https://www.healthline.com/health/anti-acne-diet
14. https://www.insider.com/vegan-diet-skin-benefits-2018-7
15. https://www.psychologytoday.com/us/blog/animal-emotions/201506/pigs-are- intelligent-emotional-and-cognitively-complex
16. https://www.peta.org/issues/animals-used-for-food/animals-used-food-factsheets/vegetarianism-environment/
17. https://www.peta.org/living/food/top-10-reasons-eat-pigs/
18. Joel Kahn, The Plant-Based Solution (Sounds True, 2020), 9.
19. https://www.choosemyplate.gov/eathealthy/brief-history-usda-food-guides
20. https://www.peta.org/issues/animals-used-for-food/

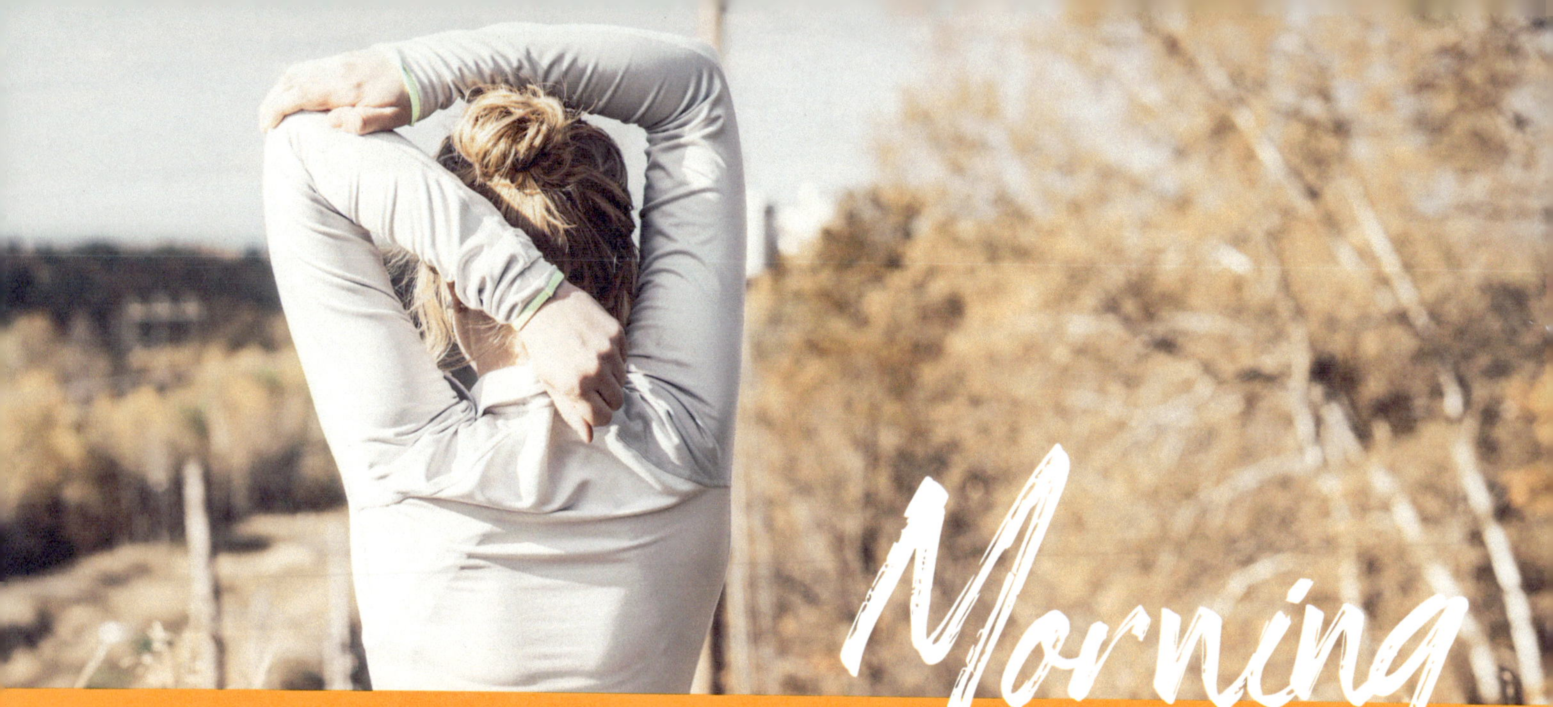

Morning

Exercise, proper eating, in addition to taking the time to be mindful and plan is crucial to having a productive day.

I am a morning person. It would be one of the first things my mother would tell you if you were to ask her about me—I am a morning person. And I remember the early mornings with my grandmother.

Every day, she would wake me up and ask me to help with her farm. We used to grow basil, tomatoes, cucumbers, green peppers, apples, loquat, watermelon, mint, parsley, cilantro and much more. One summer day in 2003 (I spent all my summer breaks with teta), I woke up at 5:00 in the morning and found her singing to her apple tree. I asked what she was doing, and she said, "I am asking the tree to give me apples again." It could seem a silly thing to do, especially to a young girl, but teta believed plants can hear us and feel our love! As I grew, I understood it more as a give and take of our love and care in which the tree gives back with its fruit.

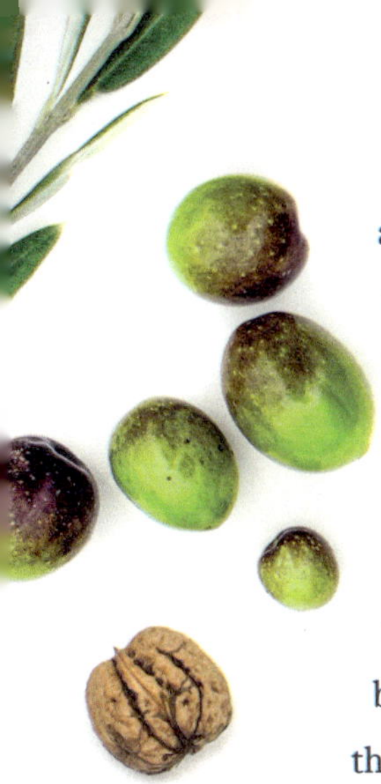

At the end of each summer, my aunts and cousins and I would to go to teta's to pick olives, walnuts, and pomegranates. The days we did that would start at 5:00 in morning and ended after 6:00 on the evening.

One of her fields was large, with very old trees. One of the oldest and biggest was a walnut tree. I remember this tree (which still exists) was the biggest I've ever seen. The walnuts that it bears can feed up to 50 people, and we used to use a large wooden stick hit the branches, making the nuts fall to the ground. My cousins and I would then pick it up give it to teta, who would peel the green flesh off and pack then the walnuts in big bags.

Teta believed plants can hear us and feel our love!

The olives we picked went to an old man who owned an olive press. We—me and my cousins—in bed of the truck, waiting for the olive oil tanks. Oh, greatest days of my life!

My teen years... well, they weren't as easy (no one's are). I started working for my father at the salon when I was only 14. I learned how to cut hair, dye it, how to do makeup, and even use the laser. He counted on me, treating me as an adult, and it was pretty tough, but it taught me how to be strong and responsible. I always suggest teenagers get a job, and learn how to be responsible and punctual—these are important lessons in life.

However, working in a salon as a teenager? Perhaps the lessons were a bit more than that. Like any teenager, I had acne (and had what we all called "baby fat," but was probably weight gain from my Hashimoto's) and wasn't happy about that after seeing all my father's clients looking the way I wanted to look! It wasn't peer pressure or jealousy—it was the way I wanted to present myself. It's important that we all accept each others' images and how we want to present ourselves, and I wanted to present myself more a woman, and less as a girl.

So, in addition to working at the salon, I also started working out at 14! Oh, yes—I was doing squats and lunges when I was only 14, and why not? I didn't read any signs with a minimum age by the gym's door—it's available for all ages! If you don't want to go to the gym, don't worry about that—do it at home! Use my routines on my website, or create your own, and start doing it in the morning (then get in the shower and go about your day). I admit that I like to have a nice butt and abs, so I'm always checking out social

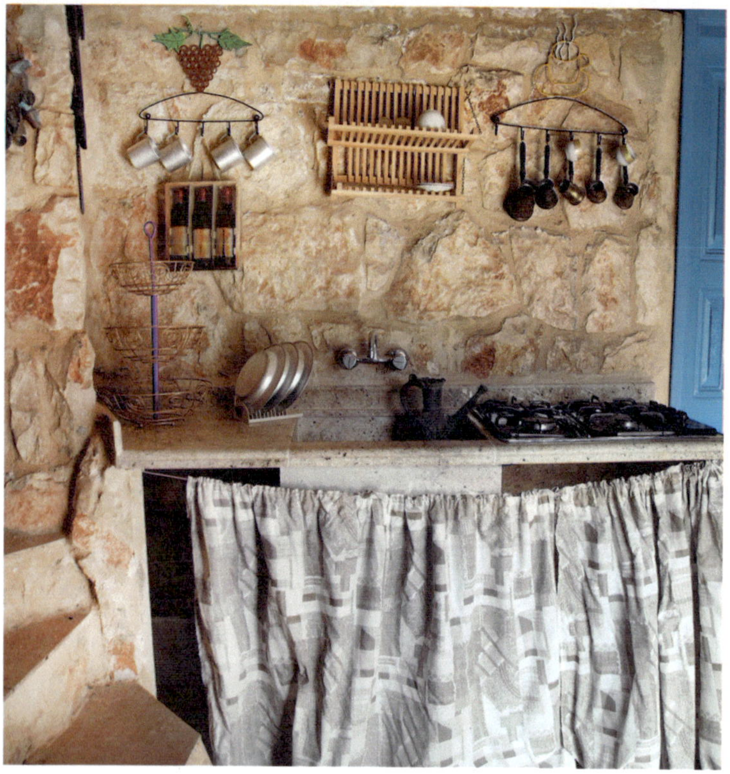

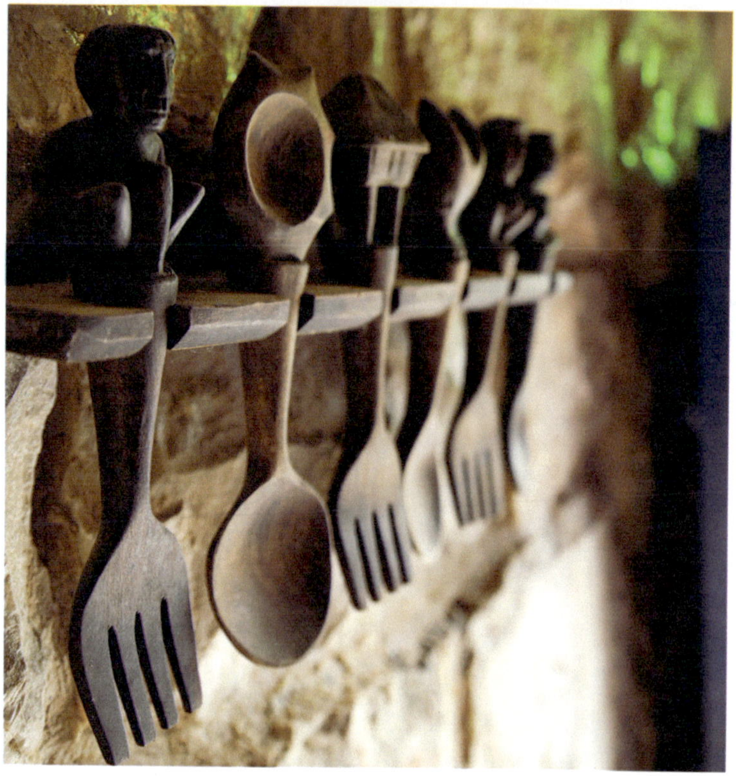

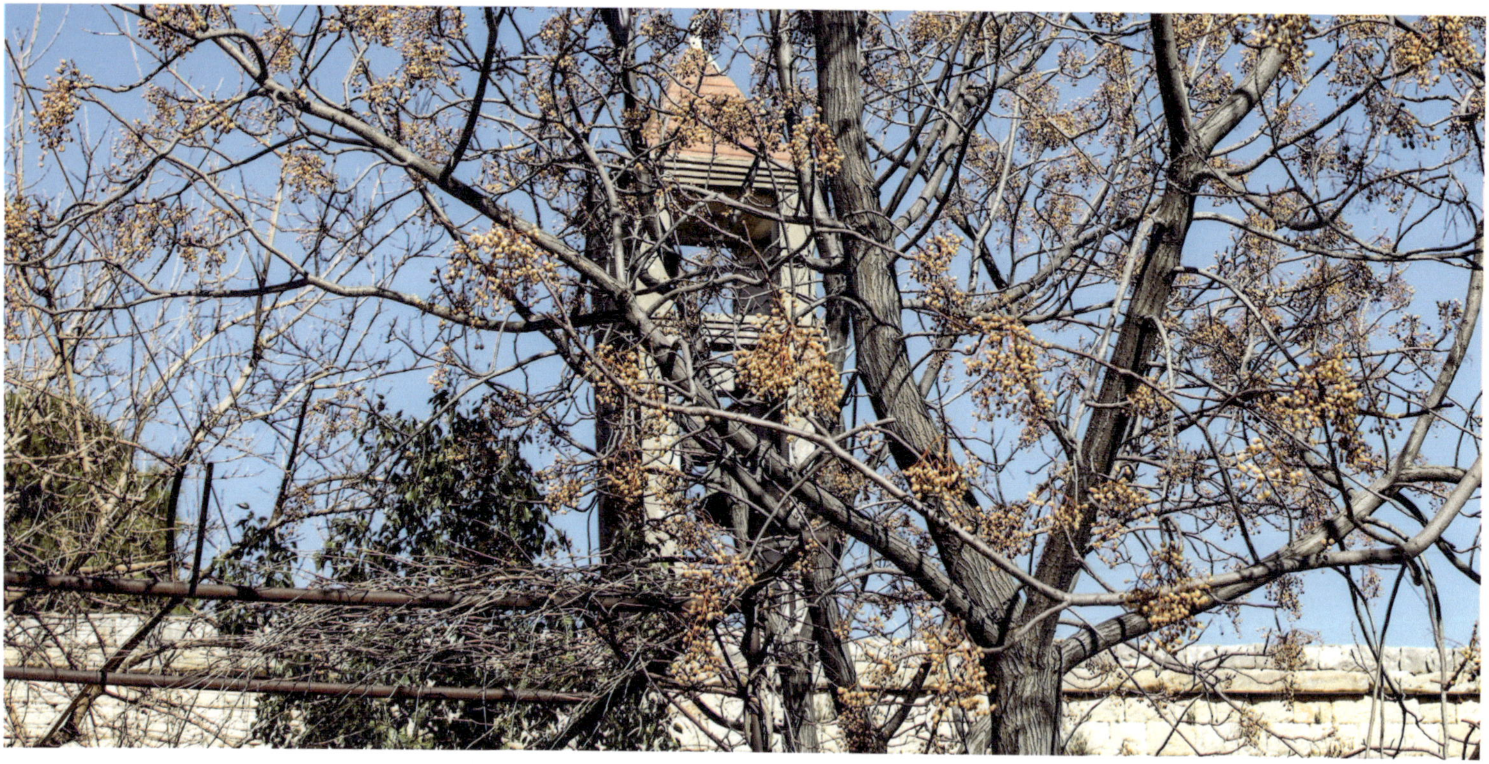

media to see what new exercises might be out there.

Now, if you have been trying to work out and haven't been seeing results, there are a couple of possible causes. Personally, I had a hard time losing weight when I was 14 because my Hashimoto's was undiagnosed. Once I knew I had that, and I was controlling for it, there was a change! You can't eat chocolate bars every day and then wonder why you keep gaining weight. You can't get lazy after school and nap for three hours, eat dinner, and then do nothing, go to bed, and then wonder why your pants are tight. If you're only half-heartedly working out, not eating well, and just sitting around, it's not going to work. If you're truly trying and not seeing results, please go see your doctor so they can make sure you aren't dealing with something (like my Hashimoto's).

As a child in Lebanon, I normally woke up to a large breakfast table of vegetables, fruit, hot bread, and hummus...

Yes, I am a morning person. I am just used to it—even in winter days, I would wake up early for school and on the weekend, I used to go help my mother in the kitchen to prepare breakfast.

Since moving to America, I can see the morning ritual of waking up in America is way different than in the Middle East. As a child in Lebanon, I normally woke up to a large breakfast table of vegetables, fruit, hot bread, and hummus (admittedly all prepared by my mother, who was up well before we were). In America, I see people who, for example, eat a bagel with some cream cheese, usually alongside a mug

Chickpea and Avocado Salad

½ can of chickpeas
¼ avocado, sliced
1 cucumber, chopped
1 tomato, chopped
¼ cup washed parsley, chopped
Juice of ½ lemon
1 tablespoon olive oil
A pinch of salt
A pinch of black pepper

This salad is quick and easy.
Mix the chickpeas, avocado, cucumber, tomato, and parsley together. Then add the lemon juice, olive oil, salt, and pepper and mix again.

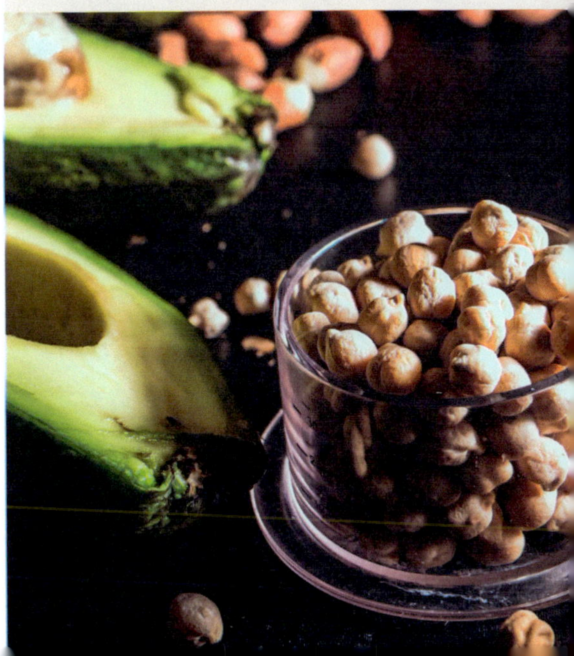

of coffee with cream and sugar.

I can understand the difference for a society that is very much "on the go," and that American breakfast is definitely smaller and faster than the table my mother lays out every morning (which would probably be considered "brunch" here), but let's look at the calories and see if there's a better alternative.

A 4 ½ inch, non-whole grain plain bagel with 1 tablespoon of cream cheese would have about 430 calories,[1] and 40 calories for a 12-ounce cup of brewed coffee with 1 teaspoon of sugar (16 calories) and 1 tablespoon of half-and-half (20 calories; 29 calories per tablespoon if you were top use light cream).[2] That comes to 470 calories, many of which are "empty," since they

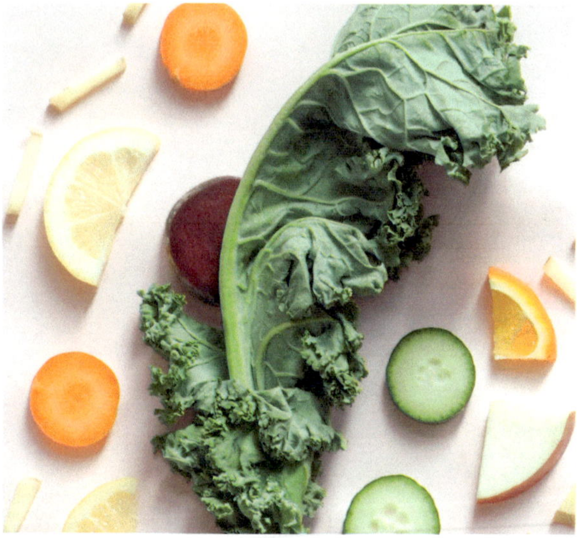

are coming from sugars and fats, and can lead to weight gain. Those empty calories can lead to you getting hungry again in a few hours

My mother's breakfast table isn't comparable (or fast), but my *Chickpea and Avocado Salad* is! This tasty, quick, and easy salad only comes to about 200 calories, very few of which are empty. The nutrient values in the salad are far better for you than the ones missing in the bagel. I know it looks like a lot of work compared to the bagel for a quick morning meal as you're rushing to get to your job, but look at it this way: What if you wake up a little bit earlier? Perhaps prepare most of it the night before (keeping the dressing aside for mixing in morning). Why are we working hard and waking up every day to go to work? To pay bills (to move forward in our job and provide a better living, or to live a lifestyle we're accustomed to), right? Your health "bills" are part of it, so you stay healthy and fit and your doctor visits are just checkups, not because something is wrong. A plant based diet will help save you from heart disease, cholesterol, various cancers, and so on. That same bagel can have 20% of your sodium

A plant based diet will help save you from heart disease, cholesterol, various cancers...

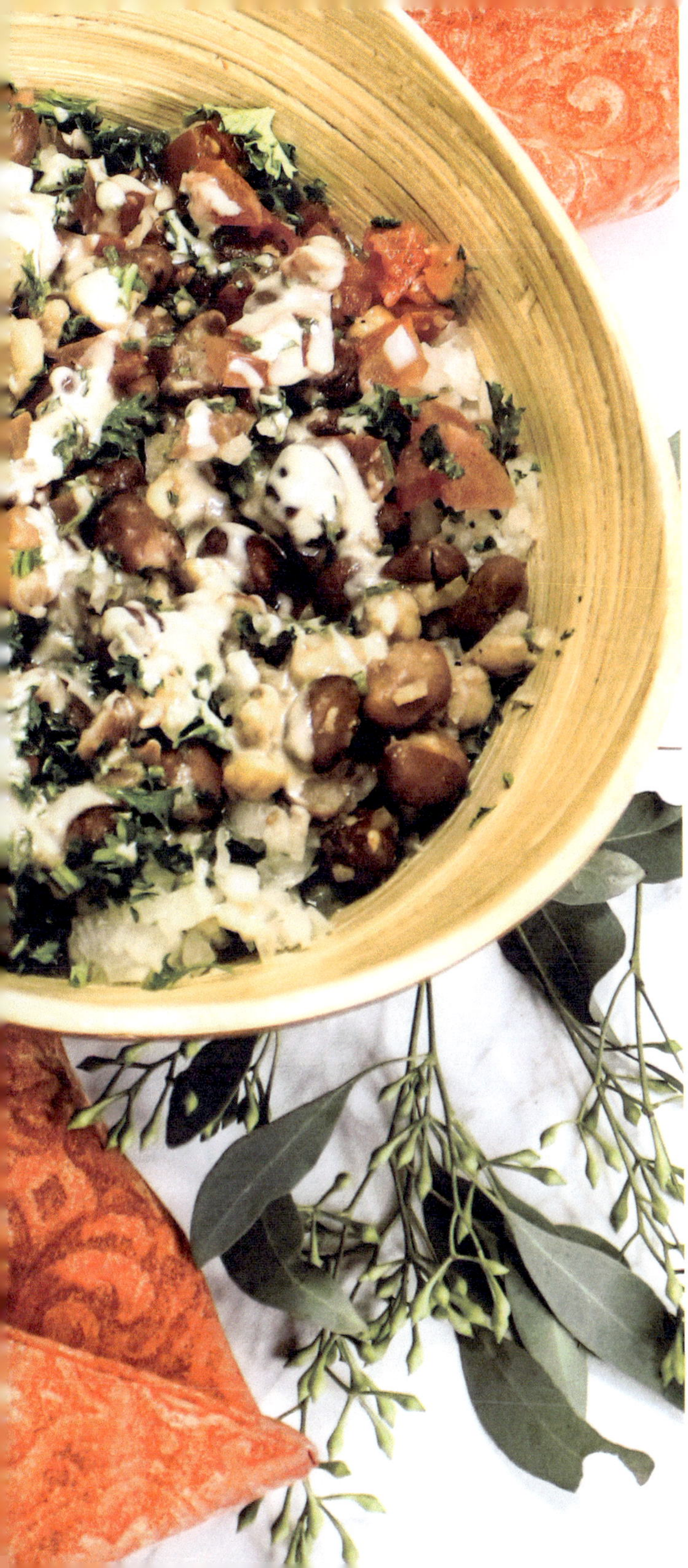

FUL MEDAMES WITH HUMMUS

1 can of chickpeas
1 can of fava beans
1 tomato
1 onion
2 cloves of garlic
½ lemon (to juice)
1 tablespoon olive oil
A pinch of salt
2 tablespoons tahini
½ tablespoon parsley

Over high heat, boil the chickpeas for at least eight minutes (taking care to make sure they don't burn). Do the same with the fava beans.

Chop the tomato, chop the onion, and smash the garlic. Then mix them both in a dish with the lemon juice, salt, olive oil.

Add the cooked chickpeas and fava beans to the mixture, pour in the tahini, smash it all together with a fork (until it has a consistency like thick ice cream), sprinkle the parsley over it, and then serve.

for the day, and that well known cream cheese and cream cheese contains 37.3 milligrams of cholesterol per ounce (12% of your suggested daily value!). If we take shortcuts to "save" time, we may only be shortcutting our health.

Perhaps you have a bit of time the night before? My almost everyday breakfast is my *Overnight Oats* recipe. In the morning you mix the soaked oats with the fruits, almond butter and chia seed, and it can be packed for school or work—very versatile!

It's worth noting that, in Lebanon, we eat chickpeas throughout the day. At breakfast, for example, we might make another dish my teta taught me to make, *Hummus Medames*. It's a bit more work, so maybe it would be a good part of a Sunday breakfast meal, or something you make on the weekend and parcel out over the week. It's tasty and gives you great energy and strength to start the day.

Of course, some people have tummy trouble when they eat chickpeas and neither of these recipes are useful. In those cases, I suggest one of the protein shakes I sometimes make. Not only are these great meal replacements, the *Kale Protein Shake* can help boost hair growth, the *Coconut Shake* can help your skin, and the *Banana Shake* is just nice and tasty! The idea behind these shakes are to help you get the nutrients you need. For example, if you're looking to promote your hair growth, then adding protein (vegan, naturally), vitamins B, C, D, and E, essential fatty acids, and (in the case of a deficiency) zinc and/or iron to your diet may help. Alternatively, sugary foods may contribute to hair loss[3], so don't add sugar it to a shake or smoothie—stick to natural sweeteners such as agave syrup (and in the smallest amount that works for you).

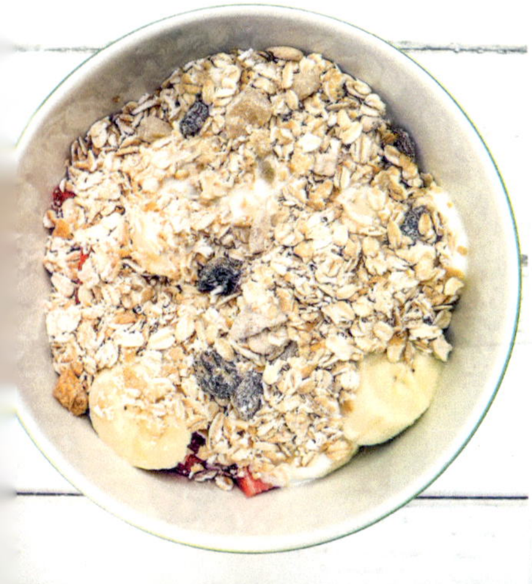

Overnight Oats

1 cup oats
1 cup pomegranate juice
1 cup pomegranate
½ cup blueberries
½ cup strawberries
1 tablespoon almond butter
1 tablespoon chia seed

Soak the oats in the pomegranate juice overnight. In the morning, mix the soaked oats with the rest of the fruits, almond butter and chia seed. Eat or pack for later.

PROTEIN SHAKES

Kale Shake

½ cup kale

¼ cup pineapple

½ apple

1 cup almond milk

½ teaspoon turmeric

½ teaspoon ginger

1 scoop of your preferred vegan protein powder

A food processor will make quick work of this, but if you don't have one, cut the fruit and vegetables so it's easier for your blender to mix. Then liquify it all in the food processor or your blender, pour into a glass and enjoy!

Coconut Shake

1 banana

1/2 cup coconut water

1 frozen banana

¼ cup pineapple

1/2 cup mango

2 cups spinach

1/2 avocado

1 tablespoon flax seeds

1 scoop of your preferred vegan protein powder

Freeze a banana the night before. A food processor will make quick work of this, but if you don't have one, cut the fruit and vegetables so it's easier for your blender to mix. Then liquify it all in the food processor or your blender. Add coconut water if it's too thick for you (or too thick to get through a straw). Pour into a glass and enjoy!

Banana Shake

½ cup water

½ cup spinach

½ cup romaine lettuce

½ lemon

4 celery stalks

½ banana

½ pear

½ apple

1 scoop of your preferred vegan protein powder

A food processor will make quick work of this, but if you don't have one, cut the fruit and vegetables so it's easier for your blender to mix. Then liquify it all in the food processor or your blender, pour into a glass and enjoy!

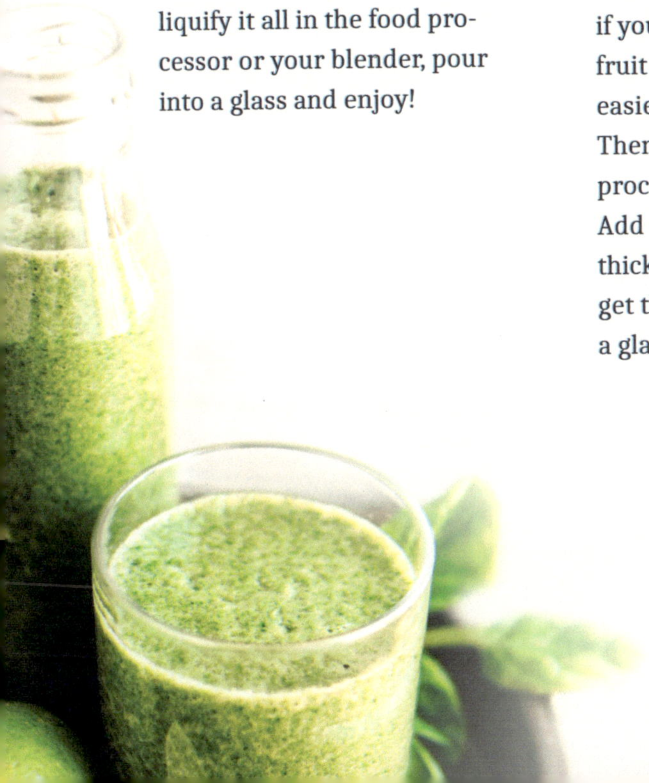

Much like the morning of a new day, adopting a vegan lifestyle has the potential to change your life. As I mentioned before, my father's health changed for the better after following my program. His high triglyceride and cholesterol levels decreased, and his BMI even went from being "overweight" to "normal." It wasn't overnight, but it didn't take that long, either. It's important to understand, whether you have health issues or not, going vegan will help you. Just keep in mind no one thing will fit everyone, so a little bit of research to help you understand what your body needs will go a long way.

ENDNOTES

1. https://www.livestrong.com/article/325712-how-many-calories-in-a-plain-bagel-with-cream-cheese/
2. https://www.livestrong.com/article/294062-caffeine-calories-in-a-12-ounce-coffee-with-sugar-cream/
3. https://www.shape.com/lifestyle/beauty-style/worst-diet-mistakes-your-hair-and-nails

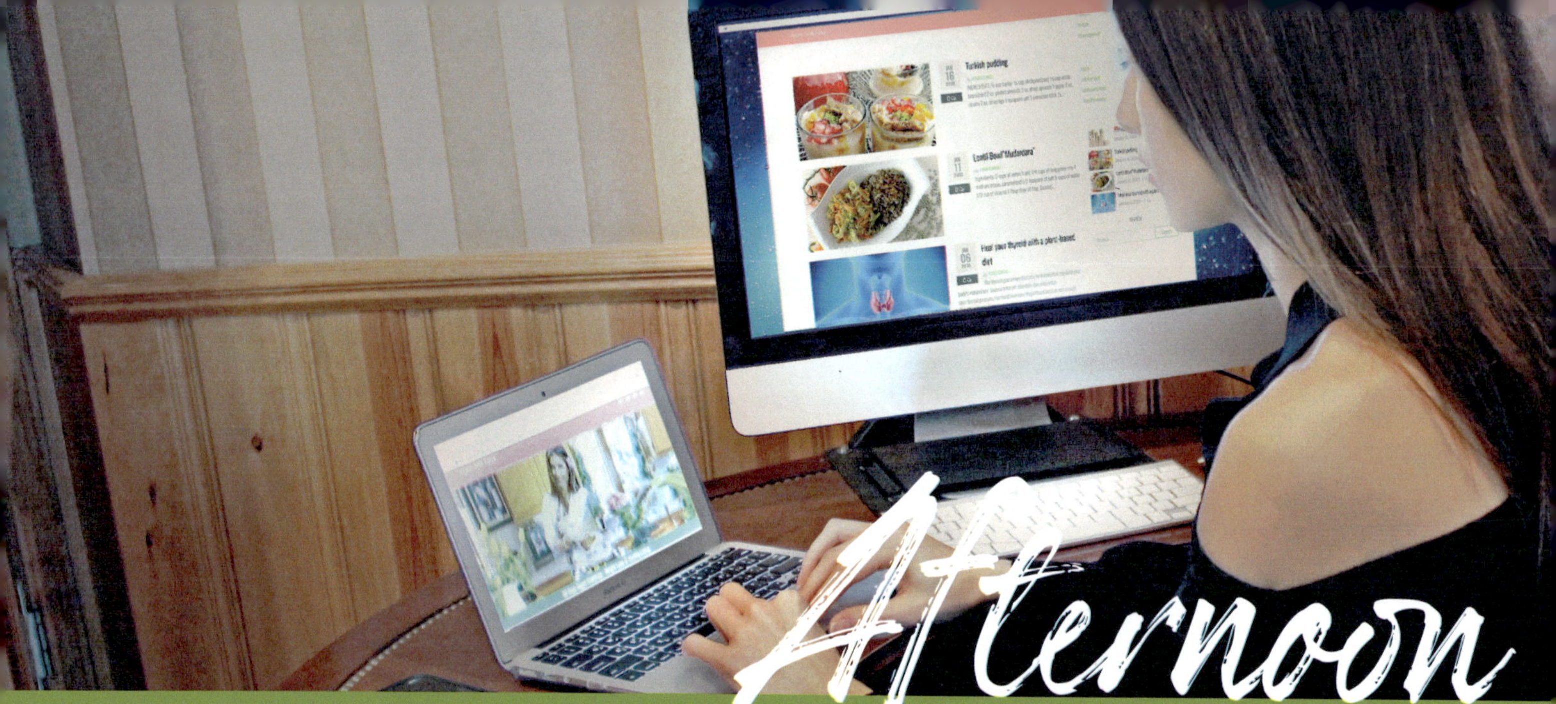

Afternoon

Succeeding in your goals can be difficult—there will be times you are tired, and sometimes you will fail. Learn from all of it, stay focused, and you will move forward.

When I was 11, my mother was coming to the end of a pregnancy, and teta came to stay with us to help out. Teta decided to prepare chicken for lunch the day my mother went into labor. She bought it, cleaned it, and cooked it. I was very young, but I knew that cats eat meat, and their canine teeth are to help them hunt their prey. Our canines aren't like that, so that meant to me that we weren't carnivores like they are. So… I stole all the chicken teta prepared, put it in a bag, and gave it to one of the stray cats in the neighborhood.

I remember teta's sandal smacking me in the head when she found out what I had done—but it was worth it!

Afternoon is a time for parents and children. Babies napping, older kids playing, and parents trying to keep up.

For some of my clients, pregnancy and motherhood have been seen as barriers to veganism. Particularly those who are pregnant or breastfeeding, there are concerns about what a plant-based diet will do to the developing fetus or the young baby. I'm here to say you don't have to worry—you can be a vegan and still ensure your baby, whether in utero or at your breast, gets the nutrients they need.

Pregnancy

Is it possible to eat a plant-based diet and still supply the developing fetus inside you with the nutrients it needs? We hear all the time about what they need to make sure their brains form correctly and so on—can you do that as a vegan?

The answer is yes!

The folks at *What To Expect* agree—"vegetarians and vegans have perfectly healthy pregnancies and babies."[1] One of the crucial things to understand is whether in utero or breastfeeding, the baby receives all of their nutrients from you, and your body is doing what it naturally does to provide for your child. Unless you, or the baby, have a medical condition that requires something different (talk with your doctor and the baby's pediatrician about your options if that's the case), you simply need to follow a healthy lifestyle to have a healthy pregnancy and healthy baby. I have worked with many clients and friends who have been able to successfully eat a plant-based diet during their pregnancies (and I became pregnant while putting the finishing touches on this book) and while breastfeeding.

Follow a healthy lifestyle to have a healthy pregnancy and healthy baby.

Your doctor has the last word in all of this (as they will be monitoring your health throughout your pregnancy), but there are particular parts of your diet you want to make sure you are getting enough of—calcium, protein, iron, folic acid, vitamins B12 and D, and omega-3 fatty acids.

If you think about it in fundamental terms, your body is building the baby, and it has to take from you to "build" them. Calcium is one of the most essential parts to be aware of—you need at least 1,000 mg a day of it while you're pregnant. If your calcium intake is low, your body will pull from your personal calcium to form the baby's and put you at significant risk for various bone

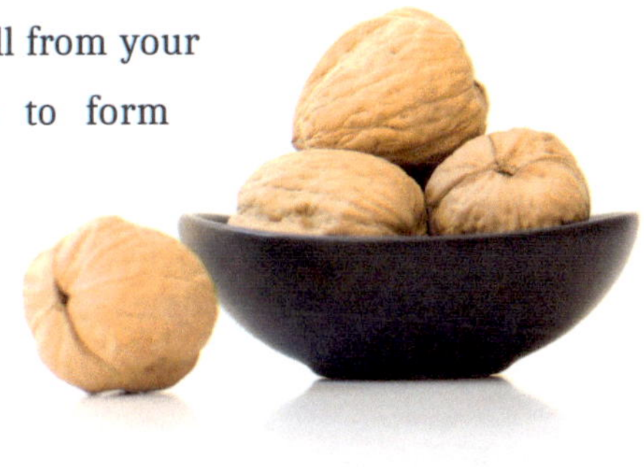

disorders later,[2] especially if you end up having multiple pregnancies and you're calcium deficient across all of them. Even if you aren't pregnant, but you think you may want to try (or, maybe it's a "whatever happens, happens" approach—no judgment here), starting to increase your intake of soy (particularly calcium-set tofu and soy milk), leafy green veggies, and even things like orange juice with calcium (just watch the amount of sugar you're taking in) will help a lot. I'd suggest drinking my *Kale Shake* on page 18 at some point during the day—it will get your calcium and protein intake up for the day (and it's tasty!).

Speaking of protein… that's, of course, vital to you and the baby. Protein is essential to the building blocks of life—our cells—so you can't really skimp on it. I don't want to go overboard about all the sources of protein you have at your disposal as a vegan—that's all in the Introduction starting on page 1—but I do have to reinforce how important protein is in your diet when you're pregnant. You're going to need about 75 g per day, so make sure to eat a lot of legumes, soy, nuts, and seeds. Chickpeas are a great option here, so my *Ful Medames with Hummus* recipe on page 16 could be your go-to for this. Or how about *Vegan Lasagna* for lunch? With whole wheat pasta and tofu? That's a protein-packed treat!

You're going to need about 75 g of protein per day, so make sure to eat a lot of legumes, soy, nuts, and seeds

The need for iron also increases during pregnancy, as the volume of blood in your body increases by 50%,[3] and that decreases your blood's hemoglobin (which is the oxygen-carrying component of your red blood cells) concentration,

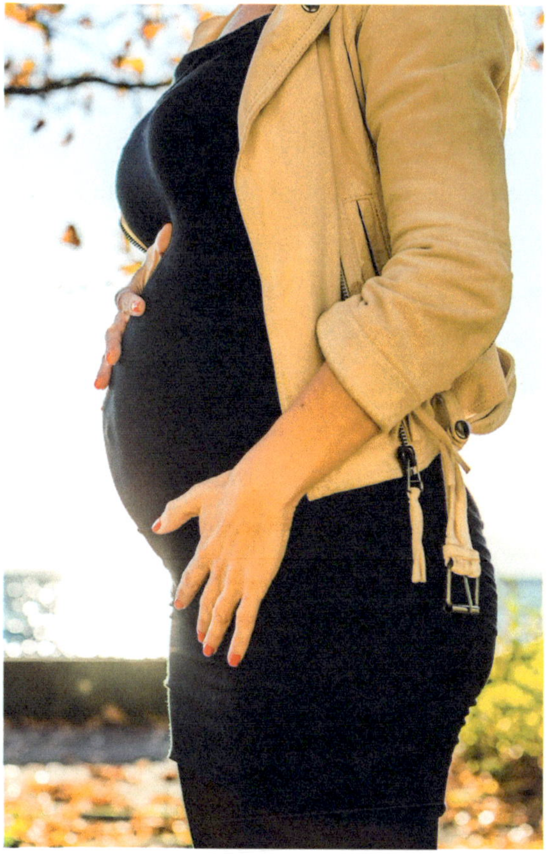

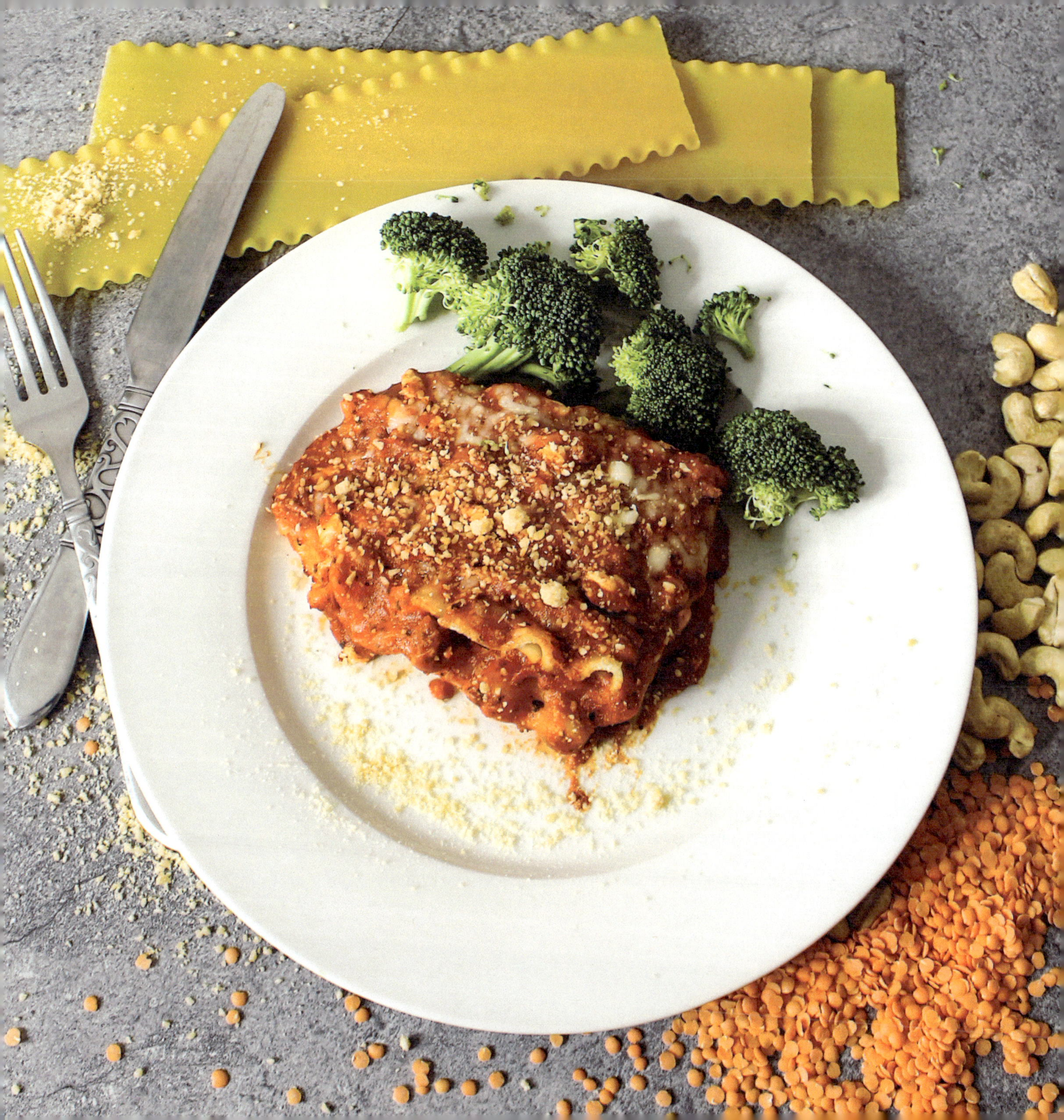

VEGAN LASAGNA

1 cup dried red lentils
4 cups water (3 at the start, 1 a little later)
1 teaspoon salt
16 ounces firm tofu
1 medium onion
1 tablespoon olive oil
3 tablespoons tomato sauce
1 teaspoon dried basil
1 teaspoon oregano
1 cup raw cashews
1 box lasagna noodles
2 mashed garlic cloves
Vegan mozzarella (to taste)

Preheat your oven to 350° F.

Cook the red lentils by placing them in a medium pot with the water and salt. Bring to a boil, and then simmer for about 20 minutes. Take the tofu, pat it dry with paper towel, and break it up a bit.

Drain the lentils after the 20 minutes and set aside with the tofu.

In a pan, heat the olive oil. Chop the onion and smash the garlic. Add the onion to the pan, cooking till it's soft and translucent. Then add the garlic and cook for five minutes.

Add the cooked lentils, the tomato sauce, and the remaining 1 cup of water and stir to combine.

Add the basil and oregano, mix well, and let cook 10 minutes on low.

While that cooks, put the cashews in the food processor and pulse until crumbly. Then add the tofu and pulse until well combined and smooth.

In a 9"x13" casserole dish or lasagna pan, place a layer of lasagna noodles (they can overlap). Spread half of the cooked lentils over the noodles, then half of the tofu and cashew mix on top of that. Repeat (noodles, lentils, tofu and cashews). Spread vegan mozzarella on top and bake for 20 minutes.

If you like it crispy on the top, set it under the broiler and watch it closely so it doesn't burn.

and your body needs iron to make hemoglobin… you can see where that's going. Your doctor can determine how much iron you need (you can have too much, so don't just think more iron is always good), so be sure to ask them once you're pregnant. You can do iron supplements, but plenty of great foods—like lentils, spinach, kale, chard—are packed with it, too. Avoid tea and coffee with your meals since they contain tannins and polyphenols, and those make it more difficult to absorb iron from vegetables. Also include vitamin C—orange juice and tomato sauce, for example (watch the sugar levels), or oranges, tomatoes, broccoli, or even the *Bazella* recipe on page 40—to help your body absorb the iron. *Teta's Lemon and Lentil Soup* on page 32 would be a great way to pull lentils into your afternoon meal.

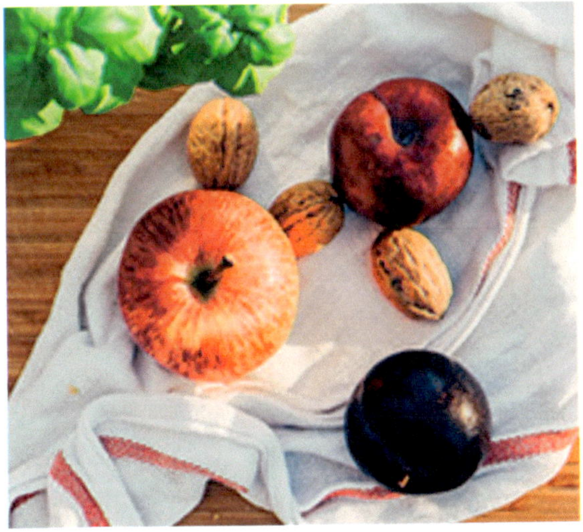

We hear a lot about folic acid and how the baby needs folic acid, which is called "folate" in food form (it's also vitamin B9). It is enormously important in building the baby's DNA, brain, and red blood cells. Not having enough means birth defects—like congenital heart defects or spina bifida—could occur, and even miscarriages seem to go up when the mother doesn't get enough.[4] On top of that, folic acid helps you break down the iron you so desperately need, too. Amazing how this all works in a circle, isn't it?

Vitamins B12 and D are also part of this. B12 works with folic acid to help with brain development, and deficiencies in it can lead to neural tube defects, too.[5] Because B12 comes from animal products, a vegan needs to make sure they are getting enough of it—especially during pregnancy. There are fortified cereals and soy milk, but definitely work nutritional yeast into your diet—it will help a lot in this regard.[6] As for vitamin D, as I mention in the Introduction, it's something we can get from exposure to the sun—but that has its own risks. There are numerous ways of getting D if you're a vegan,[7] but mushrooms, in particular, are a great source to supplement exposure to the sun. An excellent

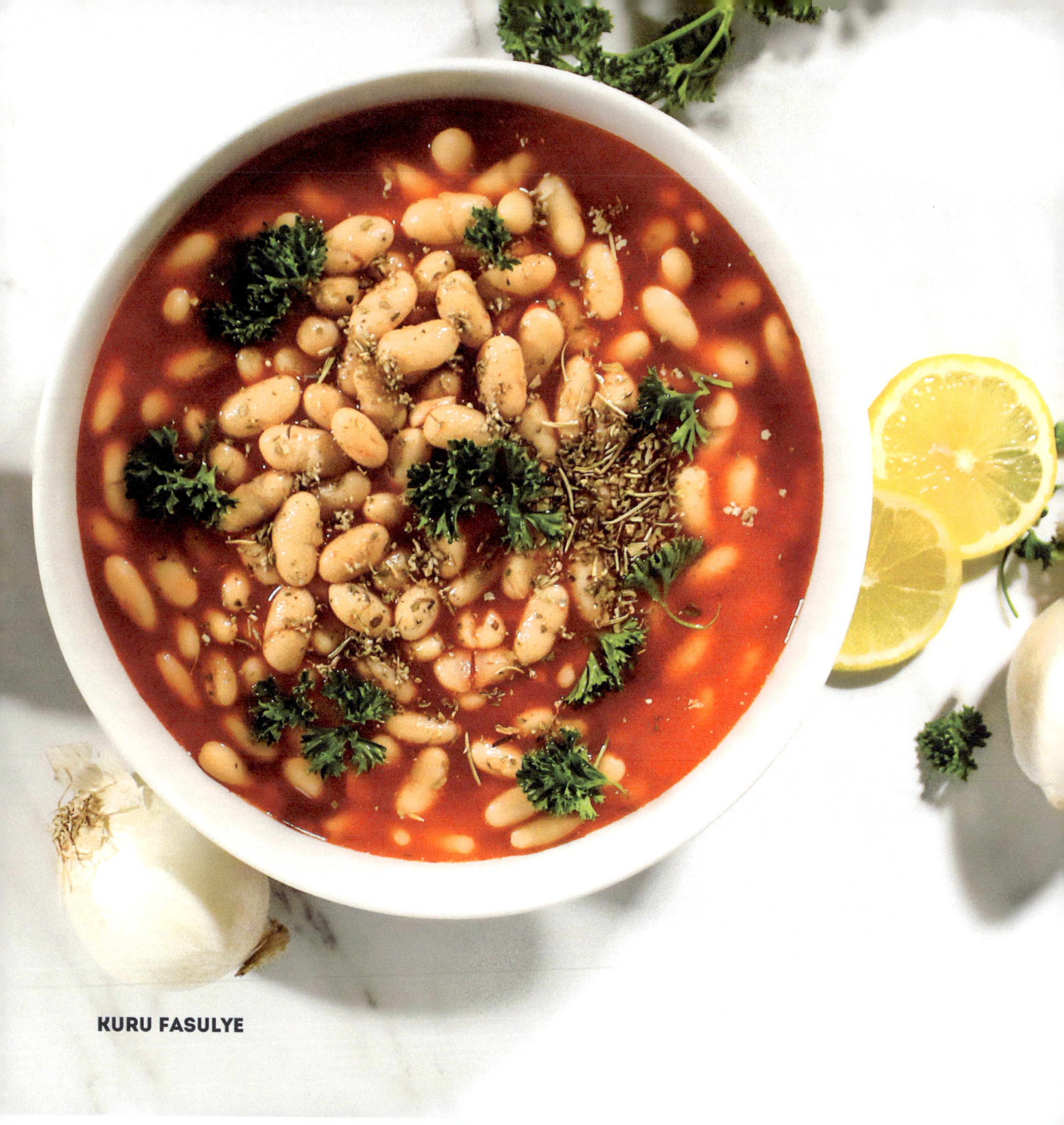

KURU FASULYE

KURU FASULYE

2 red peppers
4 tablespoons olive oil
(1 tablespoon at the start, the remaining 3 later)
3 cups of water (1 early on, the remaining 2 later)
2 cans pre-cooked cannellini beans (white kidney beans).
4 tomatoes peeled and chopped
2 green bell peppers chopped
1 cup of sliced mushrooms
4 large garlic cloves minced
1 large white onion thinly chopped
5 tablespoons tomato paste
½ tablespoon zhug* (optional)
A pinch of salt
1½ teaspoon black pepper
1 teaspoon chili flakes
Preheat your oven to 400° F.

Chop the red peppers, place in a small roasting pan with 1 tablespoon of olive oil, cover the pan with foil, and roast the peppers for 40 minutes. Remove peppers from oven and let them cool.

While waiting for the peppers to cool, gather five dishes and peel and chop the tomatoes, chop the green peppers, dice the onions, mince the garlic (if you haven't bought it minced), and slice the mushrooms. Set them each aside in the five separate dishes.

Once the peppers are cool, blend them, any remaining oil, and 1 cup water until smooth (add more water if needed). Set aside.

- On medium-high heat, add the remaining 3 tablespoons olive oil to a big pan. Then:
- add diced onions and sauté for three minutes;
- add the minced garlic and sauté for one minute;
- add the chopped green pepper and sauté for three minutes;
- add the chili flakes and sauté for 30 seconds;
- add both the tomato puree and zhug (if you're using it) and sauté for two minutes;
- add the sliced mushrooms and sauté for one minute;
- add the peeled and chopped tomatoes and sauté for one minute;
- finally, add the salt, black pepper, and white beans.

Stir and combine everything well.

Add the remaining 2 cups of water (or just enough warm water to cover everything) and bring that to a boil for a few minutes. Reduce the heat, cover, and simmer for at least 40 minutes.

** Zhug (also spelled "skhug" and "s'chüg") is a red pepper paste from the Middle East. Various American companies make and distribute it. It can be ordered online, and there are recipes for it online.*

dish for this? *Kuru Fasulye*! It will provide you with mushrooms, tomatoes, bell peppers, garlic, and onion. Sounds tasty, doesn't it?

You should also make sure to get enough zinc, since it supports your immune system. Legumes, seeds, nuts, whole grains, and potatoes are good sources of zinc for vegans.[8]

One last thing that is starting to be suggested more and more for pregnancy is omega-3 fatty acids—recent research is showing it's absolutely vital.[9] A lot of people insist the only way to get this is from fish or fish oil (including the paper cited in the last endnote!)... but that is simply wrong! There are numerous plant-based sources for omega-3 fatty acids,[10] and most are already in your diet—brussels sprouts, flaxseed, walnuts (an ounce of walnuts can easily give you your daily allowance and then some!). Some may not be, like hemp seed, chia seed, or algal oil (made from algae), but those are all resources for a healthy vegan going through pregnancy. If you feel snacky in the afternoon, fix yourself an ounce of walnuts and some seeds for variety. Just make sure you aren't eating too many nuts—they can be high calories.

If you're up to making a more substantial lunch, I suggest my *Grilled Tempeh with Vegetables and Hummus*. Tempeh is an amazing Indonesian food from soy that supplies you with quite a bit of protein, calcium, and iron while being low in calories.[11] Eating that, along with the chickpeas in the hummus and the vegetables I list in the recipe would be a great cornerstone to build your diet off of!

As you go into the third trimester, as the baby is gaining weight, you may need to increase some calories. That doesn't mean you have to sacrifice your health. Here are a few suggestions for snacks when that time comes:

» Hummus and veggies. Carrots, bell peppers, celery, cucumbers, and zucchini, are all great for dipping. Add pita or crackers if you need some carbohydrates.

» Nuts, seeds, and/or dried fruit. Mix up dried fruit with cashews, walnuts, almonds, pecans, peanuts, sunflower seeds, chia seeds, or flax seeds to have a wonderful treat. Try to get unsulphured and unsweetened organic dried fruit—raisins, cranberries, blueberries, apples, pears, apricots, dates, and prunes are great for this.

» Homemade granola. Mix oats, pomegranate juice, nuts, a sweetener of your choice (maple syrup or a brown rice syrup), and a pinch of salt then bake it at a low temperature until golden brown and crispy.

GRILLED TEMPEH WITH STEAMED VEGETABLES AND HUMMUS

2 tsps. ground coriander
2 tsps. garlic powder
2 tsps onion powder
1 tsp. ground cumin
1 tsp. paprika
1 tsp. chili powder
A sprinkle of oregano
¼ tsp. cayenne pepper
Approximately 4¼ cups of water (4 cups initially, another ¼ later)
2 blocks of tempeh (8 ounces each)
¼ cup balsamic vinegar
2 tablespoons olive oil
1 tablespoon lemon juice
1 tablespoon soy sauce
1 tablespoon agave nectar or maple syrup
Salt (to taste)
Black pepper (to taste)
Hummus (see page 16)
½ cup of broccoli
½ cup of green beans
2 large carrots
2 squash

Plan ahead—this recipe calls for the tempeh to marinate at least an hour, if not overnight.

Use the 4 cups of water to fill a medium saucepan about 2 inches up the side. Place it over medium heat and bring to a simmer. While the water heats up, combine coriander, garlic powder, onion powder, cumin, paprika, chili powder, oregano, and cayenne pepper in a bowl. Mix to combine and set the spice blend aside.

Then cut each block of tempeh into six even pieces (for a total of 12) and, once the water is simmering, put the pieces in the pan and let them steam for 10-20 minutes. While tempeh is steaming, make the marinade. Blend 2 tablespoons of the spice blend, balsamic vinegar, the ¼ cup of water, oil, lemon juice, agave nectar, soy sauce, salt, and pepper. Blend it all till it fully emulsifies (about 15 seconds).

Put the tempeh in a single layer in a shallow dish. Pour the marinade over them, submerging them as much as possible, and then cover the dish. You can marinate them for as little as an hour, but overnight is best. Flip the pieces as close to the halfway point as possible.

Save the spice blend for next time by storing in an airtight container, out of direct sunlight and away from heat. Once tempeh has marinated, preheat your grill to medium. Set the pieces on the grill and cook for about eight minutes. Carefully flip them over and cook another five minutes. You can brush remaining marinade over the pieces as they grill.

Steam your vegetables (either use the ones above or choose your own) for 10 minutes. Squeeze a lemon and add a pinch of salt over it.

Serve the tempeh with the vegetables and hummus on the side.

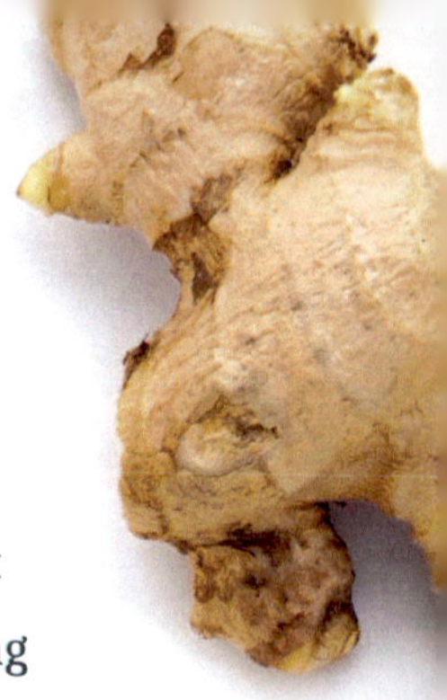

» Fruit with nut butter. A piece of apple or pear or other firm fruit, piece of fruit topped with a nut or seed butter—almond, peanut, cashew, sunflower—is a great mid-afternoon snack.

Pregnancy will physically affect your body, as you know. If you're dealing with nausea and can't stomach some of the things I've been suggesting, try toasting bread and load it with hummus, avocado, greens, or maybe a nut or seed butter—whatever doesn't sound bad at the time. You can also calm your stomach with various snacks—ginger (ginger ale, tea, jam, snaps, or the candied ginger chews are all great options), lemons (eat, suck, or sniff them), peppermint tea, saltine crackers (go with the low-salt ones), gelatin, popsicles, or even pretzels. Experiment with what works for you.

And, while not about diet, you can try to avoid stretch marks by exfoliating your skin every couple of weeks. That will get rid of dead skin. Use a hydrating mask to deeply nourish your skin. And try to keep your sun exposure to a minimum—stretch marks you have may become more obvious. Lastly, any that you have can be treated by applying aloe vera, cocoa butter, shea butter, or a blend of cucumber and lemon juice.

Mostly, along with your plant-based diet, you need to make sure you are staying active and hydrated (drink roughly 70 ounces of water per day) will also help you get through the pregnancy. Avoiding gestational diabetes[12] is important (but sometimes unavoidable), so you want to keep as healthy as possible during your pregnancy. Get out, walk, do some yoga, practice your breathing, and so on. Be sure to check out my blog at *VeganWithNour.com* to see some examples of exercises you can do to keep you active. If you're too tired and can't get going, it's okay to stop and just rest. Listen to your body.

It's not impossible, or even that hard, to be vegan while pregnant. Just keep in mind if a craving drives you to eat something non-vegan during the pregnancy, don't feel guilty—just do better. And, as I've written many times now, consult your doctor for what is right for you—we're each different, and our bodies are just as varied.

Breastfeeding

Let's start the breastfeeding section by addressing those who can't breastfeed. You are not alone, and you should not be embarrassed by that. Perhaps you can't latch, perhaps you adopted, perhaps you're trans—whatever the reason is, you may not be able to breastfeed.

TETA'S LENTIL AND LEMON SOUP

¼ cup of olive oil
2 medium onions
2 cloves of garlic
1 cup of black lentil
6 leaves of Swiss chard
2 medium potatoes chopped
2 cups of vegetable broth or water
1 lemon

In a medium pot, heat the olive oil. Thinly slice the onions and smash the garlic, then add them and cook until golden. Add the lentils and cook on low heat while you prepare the rest.

Wash and chop the Swiss chard, chop the potatoes, and add them both to the pot. Then add the vegetable broth or water and bring it all to a boil.

Check the potatoes and lentils occasionally. Once they are soft, the soup is finished cooking—turn it off and let it cool a bit, then squeeze one lemon in and stir.

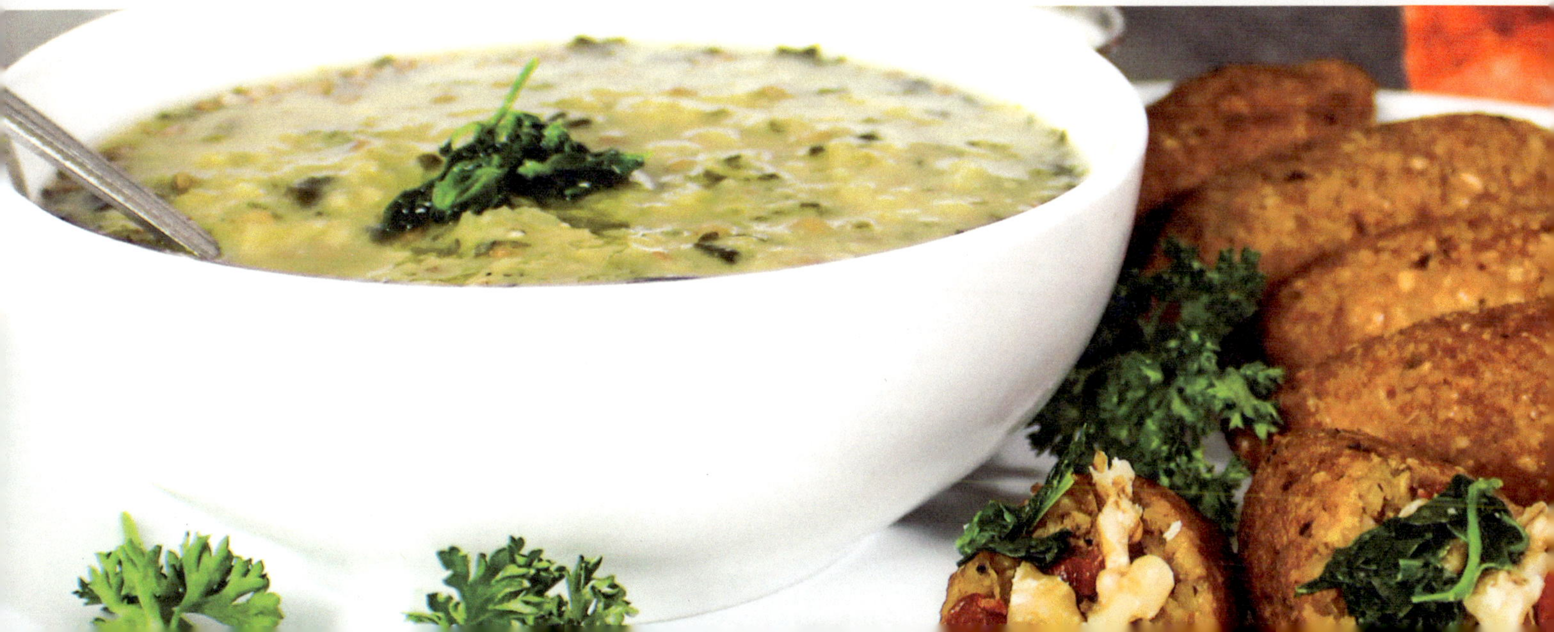

There is nothing shameful or wrong about that.

If you are lactating but can't breastfeed for some reason, then I suggest pumping (many hospitals will rent stronger pumps, so contact your hospital and see if that's an option before you spend money on buying one). If you are not lactating, or cannot lactate, I suggest seeing if you can hire a wet nurse (check with your pediatrician or maybe the lactation consultant at your hospital to see if they have suggestions) or contact a human milk bank (in the US and Canada, see the Human Milk Banking Association of North America at *Hmbana.org* for more, or contact your pediatrician) and see what your options are. If, for whatever reason, you have to use an animal-based formula, work with your pediatrician to move your son or daughter to something plant-based when they're able to handle it.

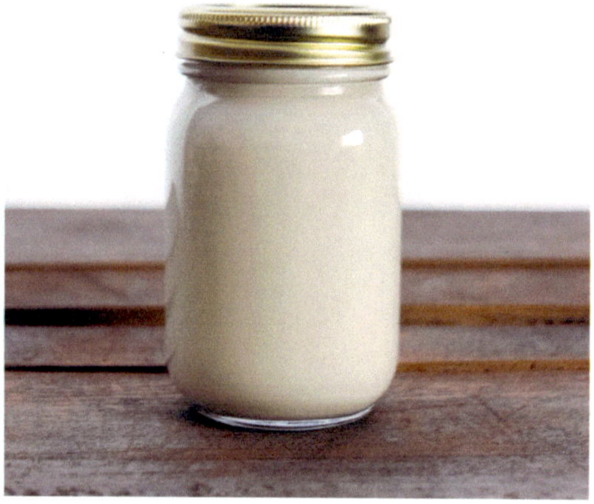

If you can breastfeed, then let's talk about how a vegan mom can handle that. As you likely know, breastfeeding is recommended for the first six months exclusively[13] (at which point you can start to introduce those flaked cereals for babies that mix with your milk), but when you stop breastfeeding varies on the baby and the mother. My mom breastfed my little brother for almost eight months, but my aunt breastfed my cousin for two years. The most important thing to keep in mind is nutrition.

You can be a vegan and still ensure your baby, whether in utero or at your breast, gets the nutrients they need

When Diane, a good friend and client of mine, sought my help when she was breastfeeding, we discussed what she needed to do to make sure she and the baby were getting the right nutrition. Emily, another client of mine, worked with me to come up with meal plans for her (she went through three pregnancies and breastfed all three babies). The key, while eating healthy, is to definitely keep up with your calcium (leafy greens and calcium-set tofu and soy milk!), B12 (mushrooms!), and zinc (chickpeas!)[14] and work with your doctor to make sure you are getting enough.

One dish I love to have breastfeeding mothers try is teta's *Bean Soup*. After my teta smacked me with that sandal and my mother got back from the hospital, teta made bean soup—my old school teta was all about health and proper nutrition, and she believed it was very beneficial. But will beans, or too many vegetables, in your diet cause your breastfeeding baby to be gassy? If you've never been around a gassy baby, it's not a smell that's the issue (they are no strangers to issuing smelly stuff from their behinds and, as their parent, you will get used to that)—it's that some have a hard time passing that gas, the gas makes them bloat, and the bloating causes them pain. So, we want to reduce gas in a baby, definitely—we don't want their little tummies causing them distress. That being said, *Parents* magazine makes the argument[15] that the gas comes from their digestive systems experiencing new things and that we need to expect it. Sure, we can remove various foods from our diets, but they also need some of that to keep their digestive systems working correctly. As the article on the *Parents* website states, if the gas is causing the baby discomfort, talk with the pediatrician and see what you can do to address it.

teach them about the health and environmental effects meat-based diets are having on us and our planet.

This book doesn't go into nutrition for your kids after breastfeeding is done—this book is about you. There are many great books about raising vegan kids out there by authors who have raised vegan kids, and I suggest reading some of those.

I will say this, though—leading by example and raising them to be vegan will make a mark on the world. Teach them about animal cruelty, teach them about how we treat farm animals (I was introduced to the movie *Babe* after coming to America and have heard that many kids who grew up with it became vegan as a result—watch it with yours!), teach them about the health and environmental effects meat-based diets are having on us and our planet. And continue to lead by example by letting them cook with you. No, you don't want the toddler chopping broccoli, but they can smash a banana or de-leaf some parsley or mint, right? Explain to them what you're doing, how, and why. By doing that, you and they will help us all become a little better, don't you think?

BEAN SOUP

½ cup canned or cooked chickpeas
½ cup canned or cooked white beans
½ cup yellow lentils
1 medium-sized onion
½ cup cilantro (optional)
3 cups of water
1 cup vegetable broth
2 tablespoons olive oil
1 tablespoon minced garlic
1 tablespoon cumin
A pinch of black pepper
A pinch of salt

Cook the chickpeas, white beans, and yellow lentils separately.

Thinly slice the onion, chop the cilantro if you're using it, and mince the garlic (if you are mincing your own).

Add the chickpeas, beans and lentils to a medium-sized pot, then add the water and the vegetable broth. Bring it all to a boil over medium heat.

In a sauce pan, heat the oil and then add the onion, stirring till it's soft and translucent (not caramelized). Add the garlic, stir for a minute, and then add cilantro and stir again. Put the onion mixture into the pot with the beans, add the cumin, salt, and black pepper. Stir.

Simmer for 10 minutes and then serve.

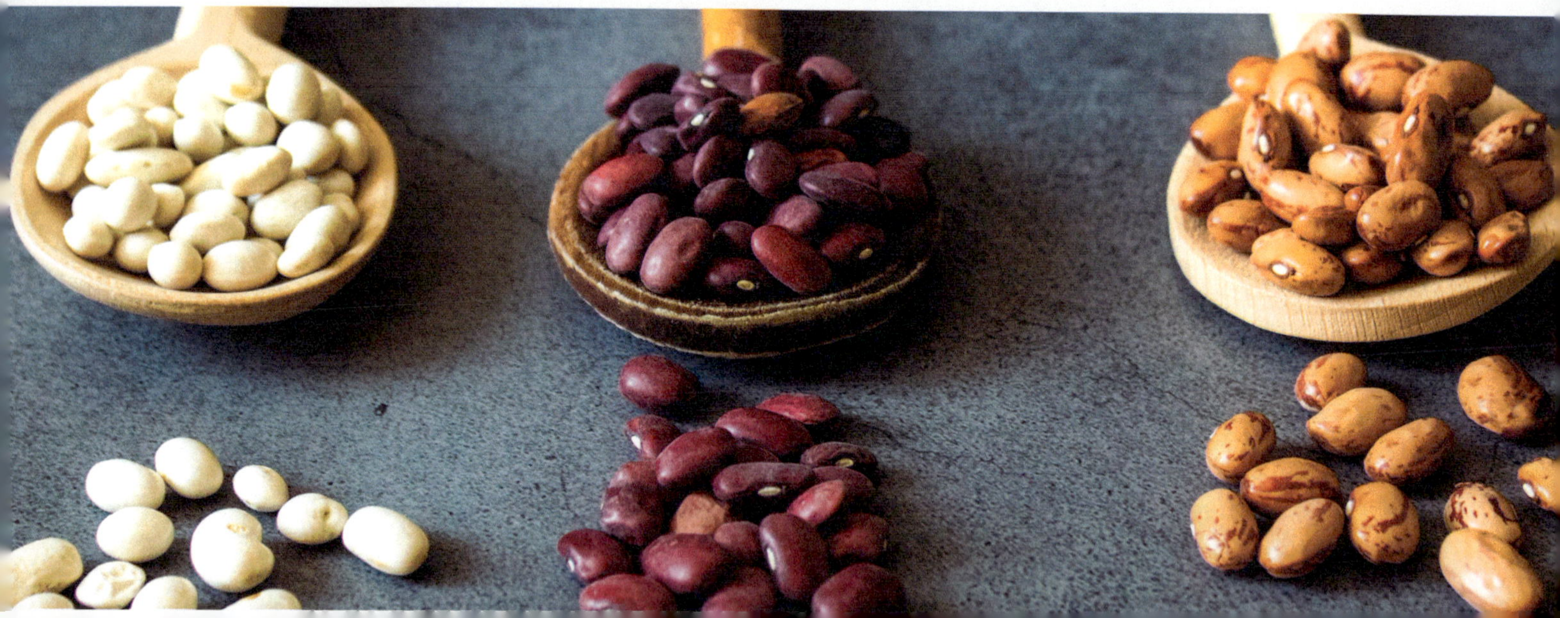

FALAFEL

- 2 cans of fava beans
- 1 can of chickpeas
- 8 cloves of garlic (10 if the cloves are smaller)
- 1 large onion
- 1 bunch of scallions
- 1 bunch of parsley
- 3 bunches of cilantro
- 2 tablespoons of salt
- 1 tablespoon black pepper
- 2 tablespoons flour
- 1 tablespoon cumin
- 3 tablespoons coriander
- Cooking oil
- 1 tablespoon baking soda

In a food processor (if you only have a blender, use that, but it might take some trial and error), process the chickpeas and fava beans for a minute or two until they look like thin bread crumbs. Put aside in a large bowl. Peel and smash the garlic. Then chop it, the onion, scallions, parsley, and cilantro and place them into the food processor. Add the salt, black pepper, flour, cumin, and coriander into the food processor and run for a couple of minutes until it's a paste.

Add the new mixture to the fava and chickpeas in the large bowl and knead with your hands until it's doughy (if it feels dry, add water and knead more).

When you're ready to start frying, sprinkle the dough with the baking soda and knead again. Let it rest a few minutes.

Set up your landing spot near the stove (a plate with paper towel on it). Then pour your cooking oil of choice into a frying pan—about one inch deep—and heat the pan over medium heat.

Scoop the falafel dough into an ice cream scoop, two soup spoons, or something similar (there are specialized falafel scoops that are easily available for purchase online if you plan to do this a lot). Don't make the scoop too large, or the falafel won't cook in the middle—you want this to be more flat than thick (if it's thicker than a really fluffy pancake, you might run into trouble).

Fry for a few minutes until it's a nice, dark brown. Take it out (a kitchen "spider"—a straining tool made popular by Asian cuisine that is excellent for getting foods out of hot liquids—is handy here, but any type of handheld strainer or tongs with a long handle will work), and place them in your landing spot. Fry as many as you like and save the dough in the freezer for another time (or fry it all up and refrigerate the remaining falafel for a few days... if it lasts that long). And, like a lot of recipes, you will have some trial and error—don't be discouraged if your first few tries aren't all that pretty (they're likely to still be tasty!).

TABBOULEH

- 2 bunches of curly parsley
- 12 large mint leaves
- 5 scallions
- 3 medium tomatoes
- 1 pinch black pepper (or to taste)
- 2 lemons
- ½ cup olive oil
- 1 pinch salt (or to taste)
- 1 tablespoon pomegranate molasses

Wash and dry the parsley and mint. Remove any stems, finely chop them together, and put them in a large mixing bowl.

Chop the scallions and tomatoes and mix them with the black pepper in a smaller bowl, then add that mixture to the parsley and mint.

Take one of the lemons and zest it into the bowl. Then juice both lemons into the bowl. Add the olive oil, salt, and pomegranate molasses. Mix well.

Taste and adjust seasoning and lemon juice as needed.

Variant: Regions and families make different versions of tabbouleh, so this might be different than what you've had before because it has no bulgur in it. Try this version first, and if you think you need something to add a little chewiness, then you can add bulgur. Start by soaking **1 cup of bulgur** in **1 cup of water** for 20 minutes, then add that to the large bowl when you put in the chopped parsley and mint (and follow the rest of the recipe).

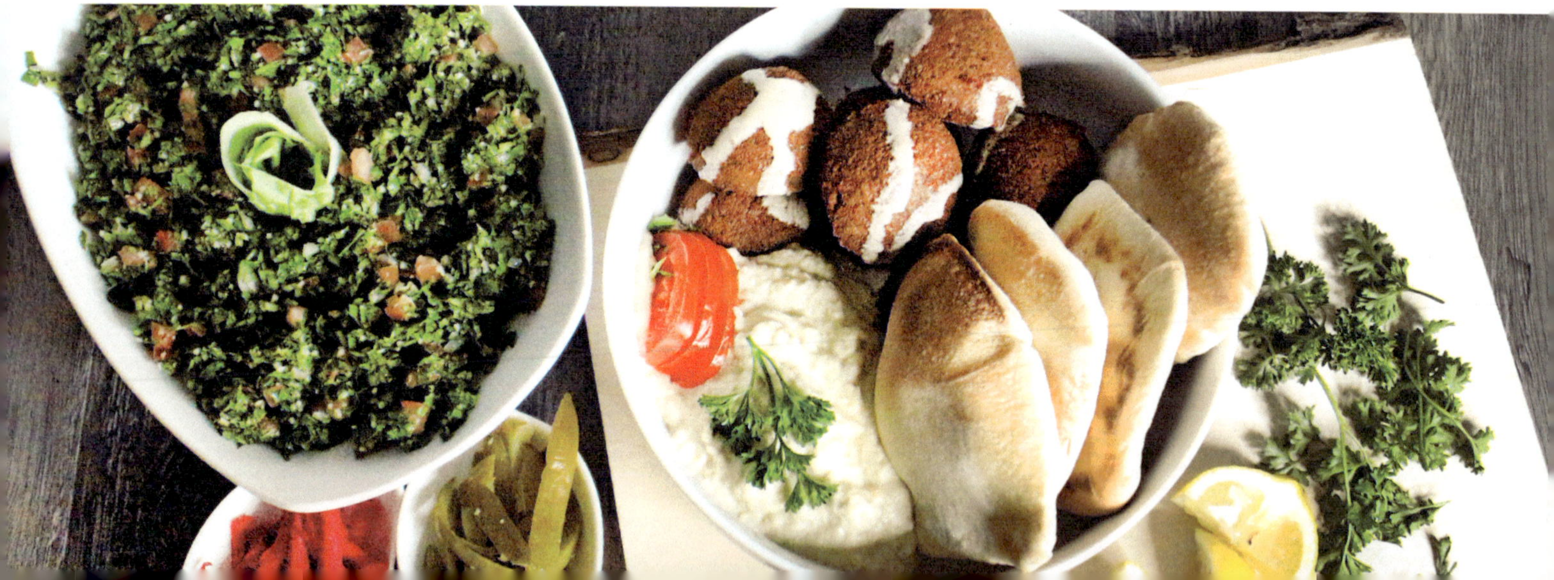

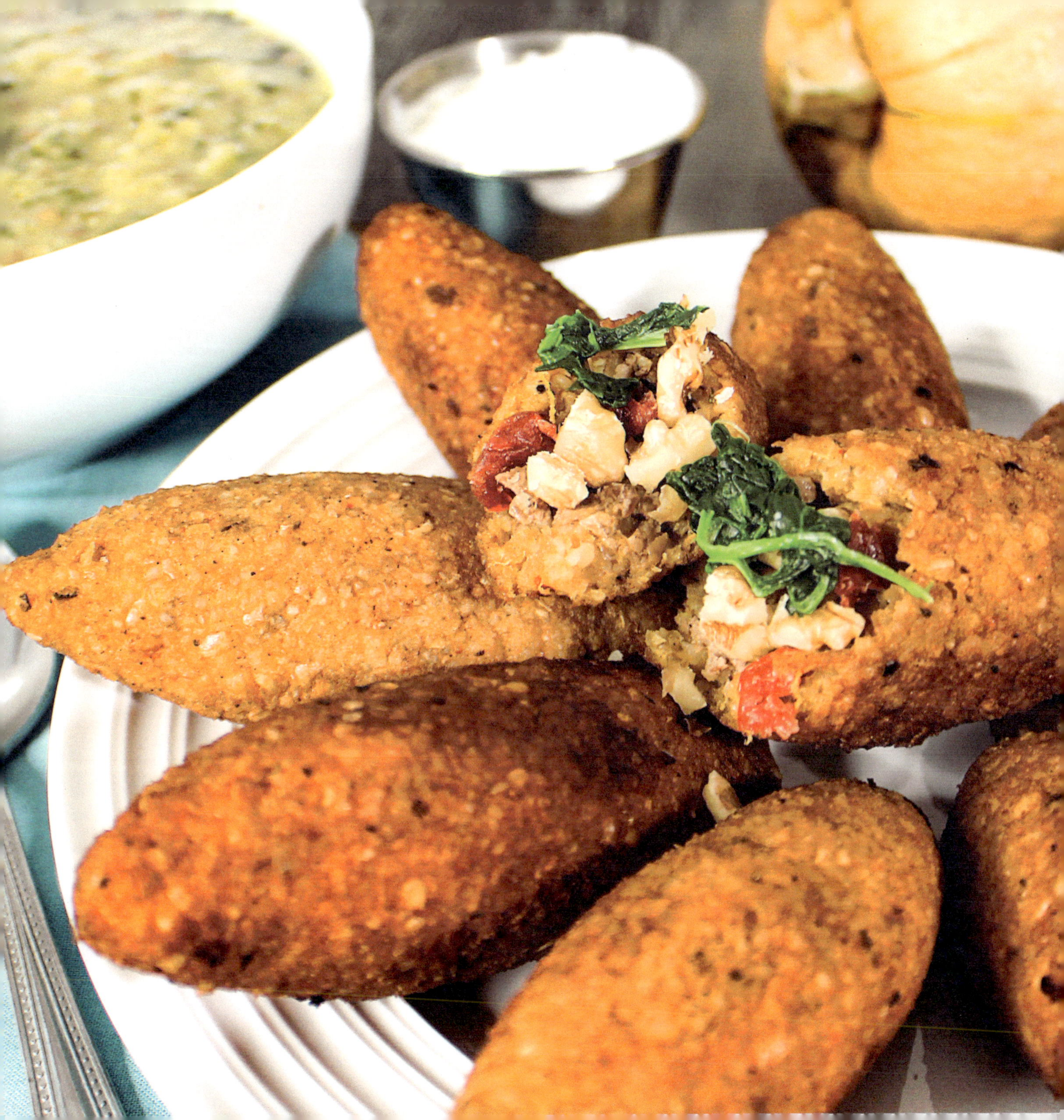

PUMPKIN KIBBEH

6 cups of pie pumpkin (not carving pumpkin)
1 ½ cups bulgur
2 tablespoons all-purpose flour
1 lemon
1 ¼ teaspoons salt
2 tablespoons chickpeas
1 tablespoon olive oil
1 medium onion
2 cups spinach
1 ½ teaspoons sumac
½ teaspoon salt
¼ teaspoon black pepper
12 cups of vegetable oil

First make the dough. Peel, seed, and chunk the pie pumpkin, then cook it over high heat until soft and tender. Drain, then transfer to a large bowl, and mash it. Zest the lemon into the bowl, then add the flour, bulgur, and salt. Keep mashing until it's all mixed well. Set aside.

Next, make the stuffing. Chop the onion. Rinse and dry the chickpeas. Heat the olive oil over medium, then add the onion and cook until tender. Add spinach and wilt it. Add the chickpeas, sumac, salt and black pepper. Once it's all cooked (everything is soft, but not soggy), turn off the stove and set aside.

Finally, cook the kibbeh. Put the oil in a large pot on the stove, but do not heat it yet. With wet hands, take about 2 tablespoons of dough and shape into a ball. Hold it in the palm of one hand then press the thumb of your other into the center, making a bowl. Place 1 teaspoon of stuffing in the bowl and close the dough over it, shaping it into an oval. Smooth it with wet fingers and place on a baking sheet. Repeat with the remaining dough and stuffing.

After you have shaped half the kibbeh, begin heating the oil in a large pot over medium heat and finish shaping the other half. Then, fry the kibbeh until dark brown and crispy.

Serve with a bowl of vegan yogurt on the side as a dip.

BAZELLA

1 tablespoon olive oil
1 cup cilantro
1 teaspoon ground coriander
2 cups green peas
3 carrots
4 cloves of garlic
1 tablespoon tomato paste
2 medium tomatoes
1 teaspoon black pepper
A pinch of salt
1 tablespoon dill weed
Steamed rice (as little or much as you like)

Put the olive oil in a pan over medium-high heat.

Chop the carrots into small pieces, peel and chop the tomatoes, and chop the dill weed and the cloves of garlic. If you like cilantro, chop it as well.

Add the ground coriander to the pan. If using cilantro, add it now and fry until the edges are golden and tender.

Add the garlic, peas, and carrots to the pan. Stir occasionally.

When the peas and carrots are cooked (not mushy), add the tomatoes, tomato paste, black pepper, salt, and dill weed. Keep stirring till it's well mixed.

Serve it with the steamed rice.

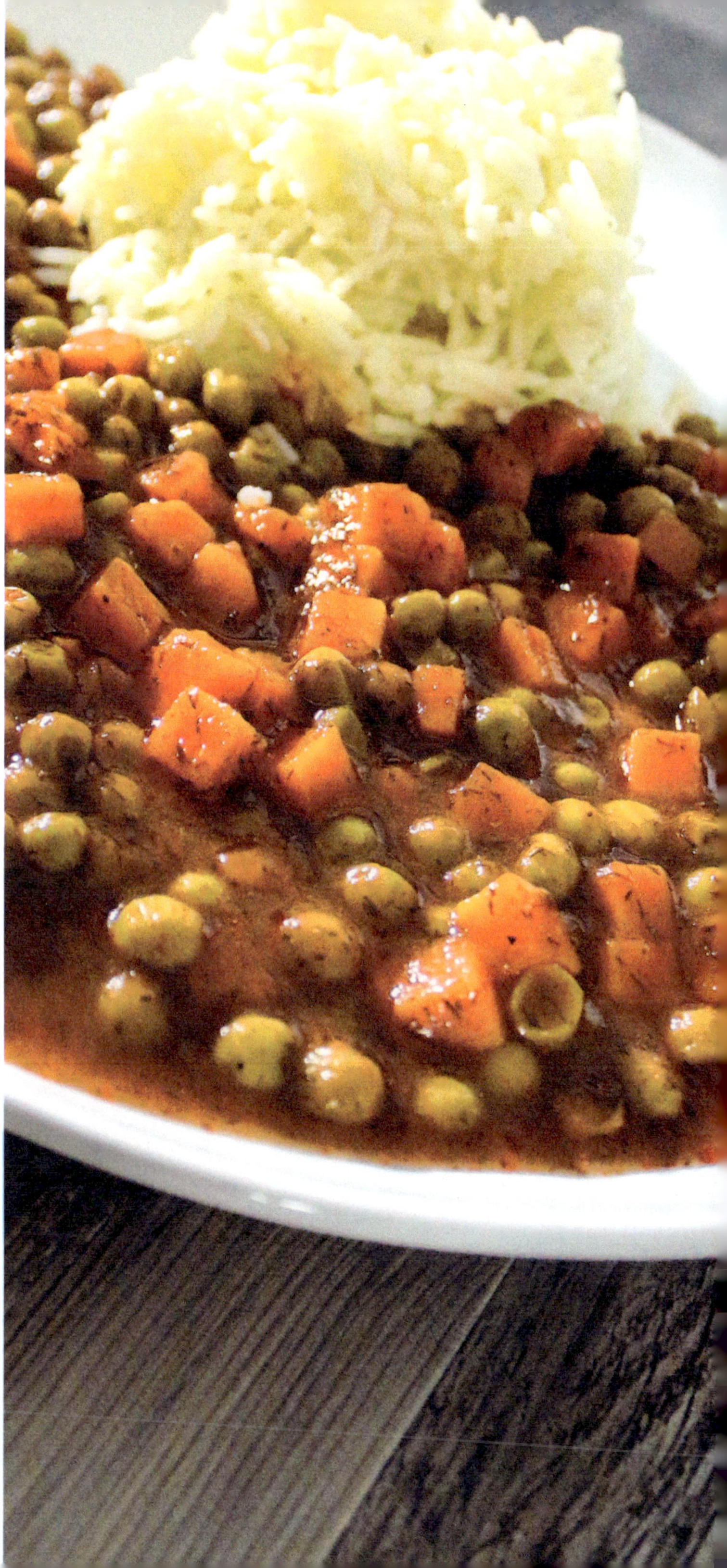

ENDNOTES

1. https://www.whattoexpect.com/pregnancy/diet/eating-vegetarian-vegan-during-pregnancy/
2. https://www.ncbi.nlm.nih.gov/pmc/articles/PMC3354840/
3. https://www.whattoexpect.com/pregnancy/anemia/
4. https://www.whattoexpect.com/pregnancy/pregnancy-health/folic-acid-during-pregnancy/
5. https://www.aafp.org/afp/2011/0615/p1425.html
6. https://www.healthline.com/nutrition/nutritional-yeast
7. https://www.healthline.com/health/vegan-vitamin-d
8. https://www.healthline.com/nutrition/best-foods-high-in-zinc
9. https://www.ncbi.nlm.nih.gov/pmc/articles/PMC3046737/
10. https://www.healthline.com/nutrition/7-plant-sources-of-omega-3s
11. https://www.healthline.com/nutrition/tempeh
12. https://www.whattoexpect.com/pregnancy/pregnancy-health/gestational-diabetes/
13. https://www.cdc.gov/breastfeeding/faq/index.htm#how-long
14. https://www.whattoexpect.com/pregnancy/diet/eating-vegetarian-vegan-during-pregnancy/
15. https://www.parents.com/baby/care/gas/foods-that-cause-gas-in-babies/

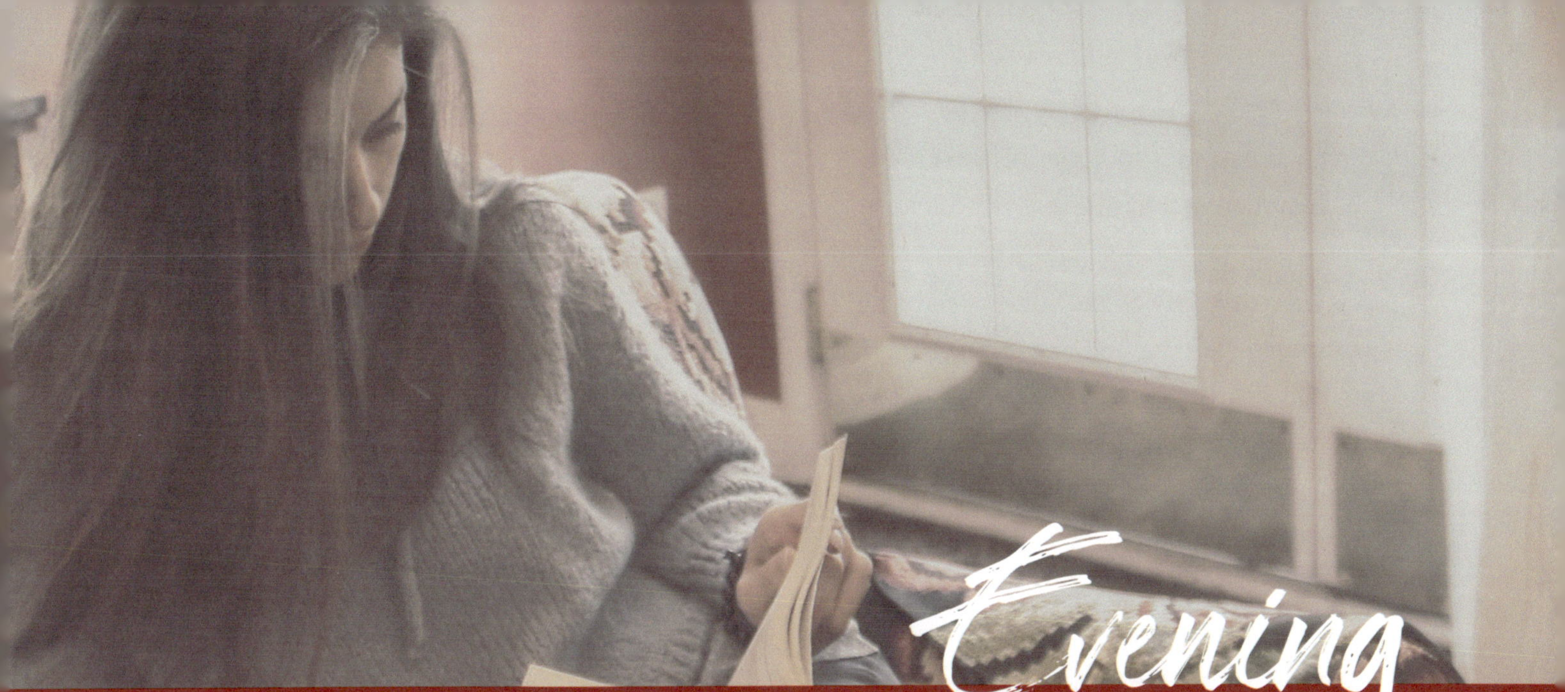

Evening

Let your soul thrive with on hope and faith, and look forward to the coming day and its challenges.

The word "evening" can mean many things to different people. In Lebanon, we would be done with our large meal early in the evening, leaving time for family and friends. In other places (especially in the United States), the evening is just when everyone is getting home and starting to think about what to have for dinner. Many cultures also see "evening" as a metaphor for growing older.

Dinner

Since coming to America, I've found dinner is where a lot of improvement can be made in our diets. We can use dinnertime to not just be a traditional gathering of family and friends, but also to introduce healthy, yummy dishes and introduce those we love to new foods.

A study from 2014 found "Cooking dinner frequently at home is associated with consumption of a healthier diet whether or not one is trying to lose weight."[1] Yes, cooking dinner can be more difficult and time-consuming, but with some planning and help from your partner and the rest of the family, it doesn't need to be—and it's going to be healthier for you and your family (and likely less costly). That doesn't mean you shouldn't go out to eat, it just means do it less often.

When we think of the more significant health issues many of us face as we get older, I think using dinner to help us rethink our diets help. Cardiovascular disease, diabetes, and cancer are three of the ones that a plant-based diet can help us reduce our risks of (but, keep in mind, some of us have various genetic and hereditary disorders that may complicate this, so always discuss this with your doctor first).

One thing that first comes to mind in dealing with heart disease is cholesterol. I always tell my father (who has had to deal with high cholesterol levels), family, and friends: the less cholesterol the better. If your blood has too much cholesterol, it coats the walls of your arteries, which ends up restricting blood flow. Cholesterol is only found in animal-based food products, not plants—but plants can contain fat, and that fat can affect your cholesterol levels.[2]

So, what are tasty dishes to serve up for dinner when you have a focus on cholesterol levels? Coming from the Middle East, I immediately think of lentils! Yes, other beans and legumes and nuts are great[3] (just watch the fat content of things like cashews when you're dealing with high cholesterol, and watch the calorie count on nuts). Something like my *Lentil Bowl* or Teta's Red Mujaddara are great Lebanese-style dishes, but for something quick, you could do my *Middle Eastern Lentil Tacos*, and what about a *Vegan Lasagna*—with lentils, tofu, and cashews—when you're entertaining?

Cardiovascular disease, diabetes, and cancer are three of the ones that a plant-based diet can help us reduce our risks

Also, when I think of dishes that would fit this category, eggplant comes to mind![4] One of my favorite low-calorie dinners of all time is my *Eggplant Mutabbal Bowl*.

Those are all lovely, yummy dishes for you to try with your family and friends, and if they help lower a loved one's cholesterol levels, and make their heart healthier, then that's even better, right?

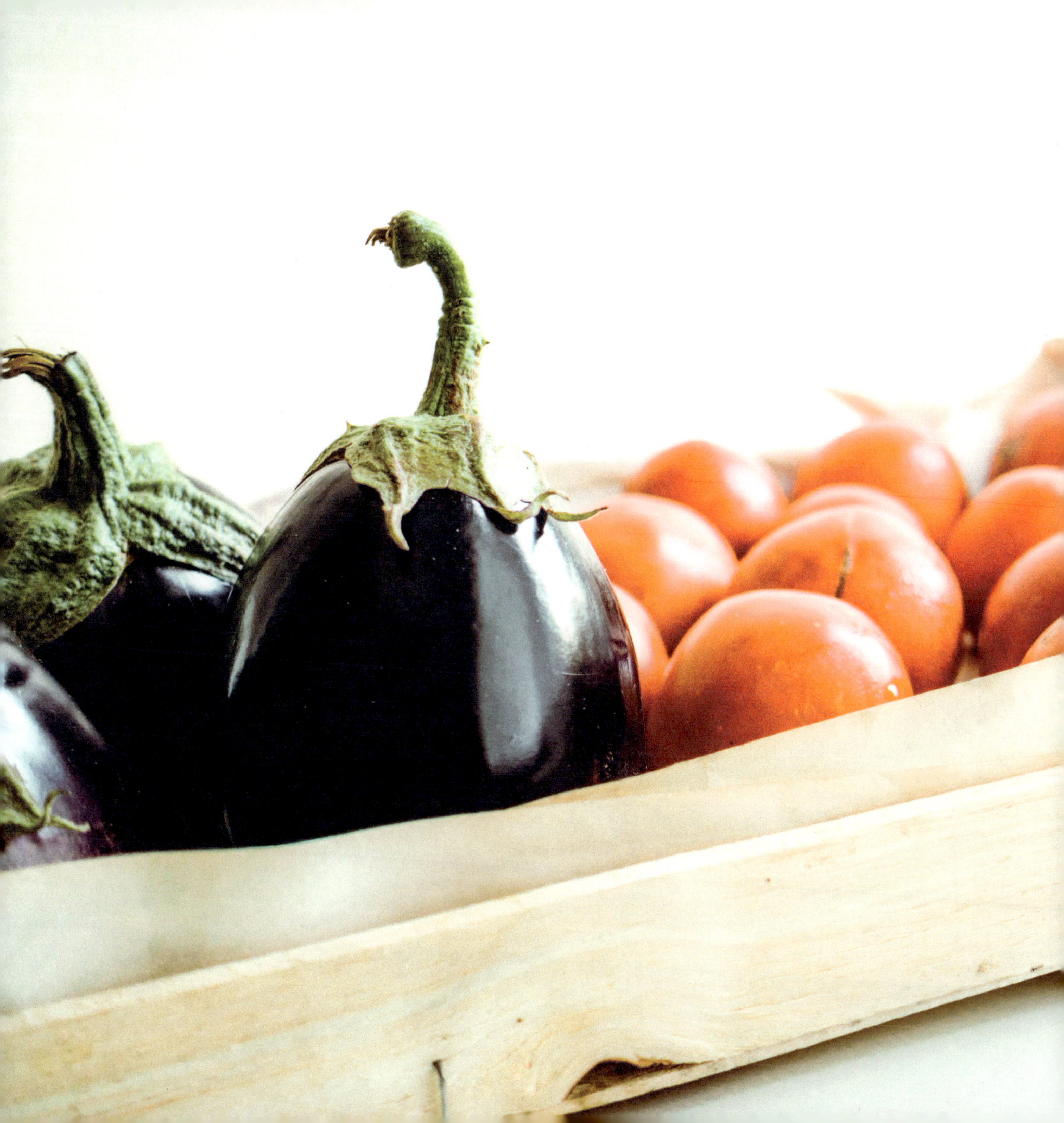

EGGPLANT MUTABBAL BOWL

1 large eggplant
2 tbsp. tahini
2 garlic cloves minced
pinch of salt
2 tbsp. lemon juice

Preheat the oven to 400° F and bake the eggplant (whole) for 35 minutes.

Once the eggplant is cool to the touch, peel the skin, and remove the stem. Put the cleaned eggplant in a bowl and smash it real good. Then add the tahini, lemon, and salt.

Mix well and serve with your favorite side salad.

You might have had mutabbal before but called "baba ghanoush." They're similar but different, and different enough that they shouldn't be confused. Baba ghanoush doesn't use tahini at all and is mixed with tomato, onions, and so on.

LENTIL BOWL

1 cup of lentils
2 cups of water
½ cup of onions
½ cup of green and red peppers
½ cup of cucumbers
½ cup of radishes
½ cup of pomegranate
¼ cup of mint
½ large lemon
½ tablespoon ginger
½ teaspoon ground turmeric
½ teaspoon salt
1 tablespoon extra-virgin olive oil
Freshly ground black pepper

Put the lentils in a pot and add the water (add more if it doesn't cover all the lentils). Bring to a rapid simmer, then bring it down to a gentle one (only a few bubbles and some movement in the lentils). Simmer them uncovered for 20-30 minutes, adding water if necessary.

While the lentils simmer, chop the onions, peppers, cucumbers, radishes, and mint. You can add or remove vegetables as you want—this is just how I prefer mine. Set them all aside.

Once the lentils are tender (not mushy) and no longer crunchy, they're cooked. Drain and set aside to cool.

While the lentils cool, juice the lemon and grate the ginger into a bowl. Add the turmeric, salt, olive oil, and black pepper (to taste).

Once the lentils are cool, mix it all together and enjoy.

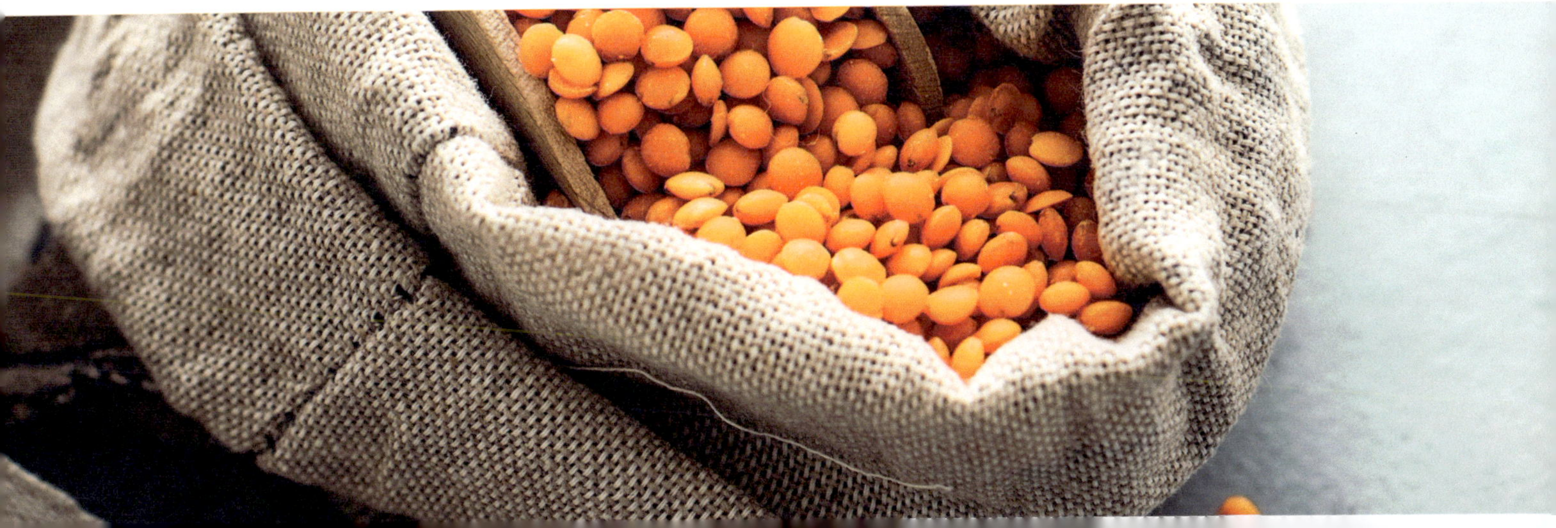

Diabetes is a challenge when it comes to a diet. We've all heard of it. Type 1 diabetes, which some children have and outgrow (some don't), is a chronic condition where the pancreas produces no or almost no insulin (which is used by our body to break down the sugar glucose and convert it into energy). Type 2 (sometimes referred to as "adult-onset diabetes" because it's usually caused by a poor diet, a lack of exercise or other health issues) is when the body is unable to use the insulin it is producing because your body has become resistant to the work the insulin is doing.

I still remember my old principal, Andrée, from elementary school. She has, sadly, passed away. She was French, and loved food—but couldn't eat it because of her diabetes. She wouldn't participate in school functions that included food (Christmas or Easter, for example). I walked into her office once, just before Christmas, and she was drinking artichoke root water. She would pick artichokes from a garden near our school, boil the roots, and drink the water. When I asked about it, she explained artichoke help lower blood sugar. It's looking more and more like that's right—artichokes and artichoke leaf extract might have a positive effect on blood sugar (it's still not known why, however).[5]

It's challenging to find dishes that are suitable for everyone, but if you're vegan and cooking for a diabetic (either yourself or others), one Lebanese dish I love that works in this case is a delightful stew called *Bazella*. Traditionally, this would be served with steamed white rice (which, if you aren't diabetic, you may want to try), but in this case, I suggest something like wild, basmati, or brown rice (in moderation), or skip the rice altogether and serve on a beautiful bed of cooked quinoa.[6]

Eating a plant-based diet, but focusing on vegetables to control the sugar, should mean your blood sugar will get better!

Eating a plant-based diet, but focusing on vegetables to control the sugar, should mean your blood sugar will get better! We can't stop type 1 (yet), but we can help regulate both types through better eating, and we can stop type 2 before it happens (and in a few cases, we might even be able to reverse it; again, always talk with your doctor about your health and its needs).

And then there is cancer.

MIDDLE EASTERN LENTIL TACOS

2 cups red lentils
4 cups water
1 white onion
2 garlic cloves
¼ head of lettuce
1 jalapeño
1 avocado
1 tablespoon olive oil
¼ cup of vegetable broth (or water)
1 tablespoon chili powder
¼ teaspoon garlic powder
¼ teaspoon onion powder
¼ teaspoon crushed red pepper flakes
½ teaspoon paprika
1½ teaspoons ground cumin
1 teaspoon salt
1 teaspoon black pepper
1 cup corn (fresh or frozen)
3 hard taco shells

Put the lentils in a pot and add the water (add more if it doesn't cover all the lentils). Bring to a rapid simmer, then bring it down to a gentle one (only a few bubbles and some movement in the lentils). Simmer them uncovered for 20-30 minutes, adding water if necessary.

While the lentils simmer, dice the onion finely, mince the garlic (if you haven't bought it minced), shred the lettuce, slice the jalapeño and avocado. Set each aside separately.

Then, in a small bowl, mix the chili powder, garlic powder, onion powder, red pepper flakes, paprika, cumin, salt, and black pepper. Set aside.

Once the lentils are tender (not mushy) and no longer crunchy, they're cooked. Drain and set aside.

After the lentils are cooked, place a large pan over medium high heat, sweat the onion in the oil. Cook for four to five minutes, stirring frequently, until the onion is translucent. Add both the garlic and the spice mixture. Cook for another minute or so, still stirring frequently—and don't burn it.

Add the lentils, stirring to combine, and then add the vegetable broth. Gently mash the lentils with a fork until they start to look suitable for a taco filling. Cook another few minutes to make sure everything is heated through. If the lentils start to dry out, add another tablespoon or two of vegetable broth or water and mix.

If your corn is frozen, prepare it now.

Place the cooked lentil mixture in the taco shells. Add the shredded lettuce, avocado, corn, and jalapeños on top. Serve with a side salad and save the rest for another day.

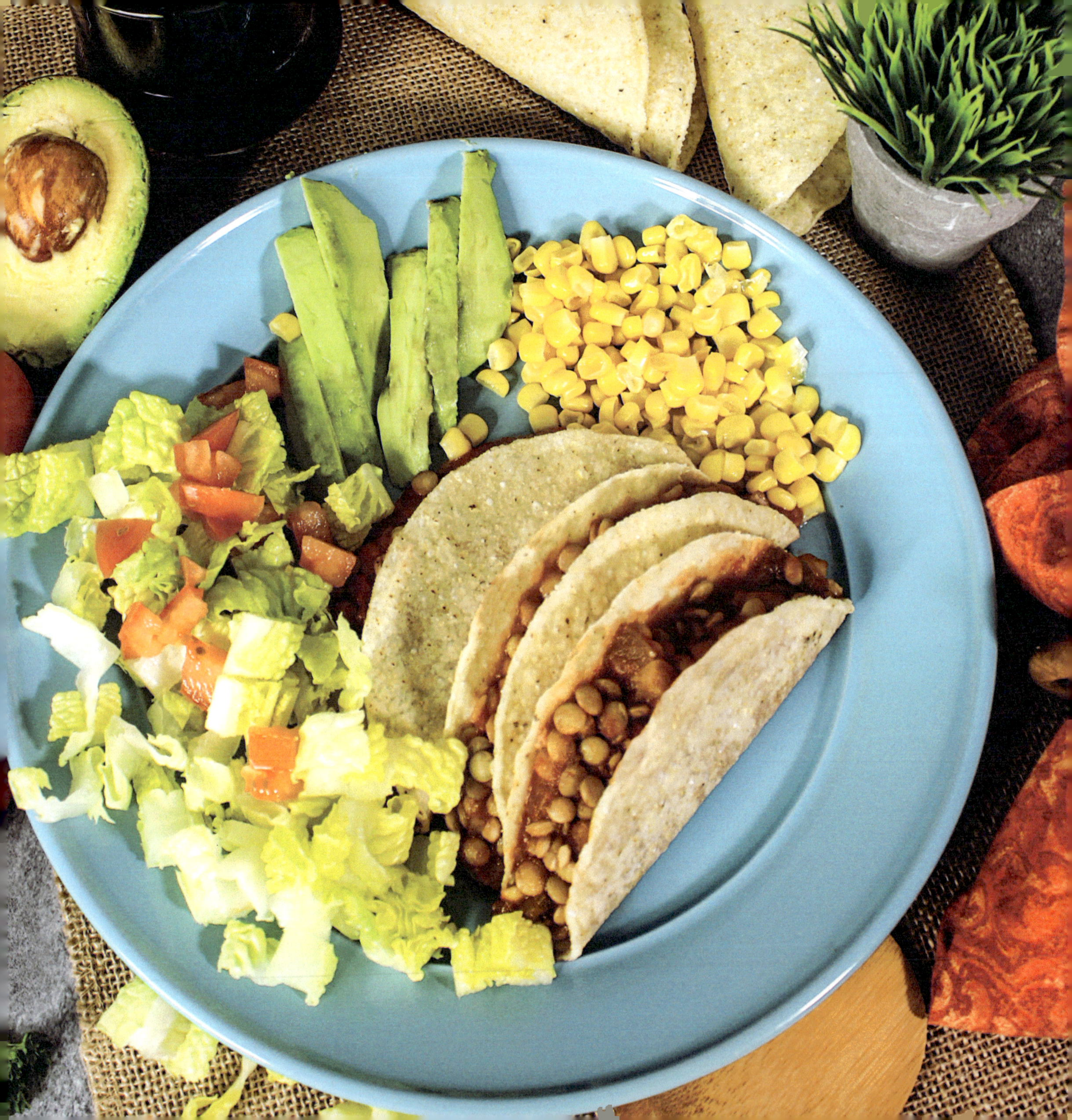

TETA'S RED MUJADDARA

1 cup red lentils
½ cup bulgur
3 onions
½ cup olive oil
2 cups water
A pinch of salt

Rinse the lentils and bulgur separately, setting them aside in separate dishes.

Slice the onions thin. Put the olive oil in a pot over high heat, and add the onions. Stir them continuously until they are caramelized and a dark brown (*dark brown—not burnt!*) color. Then add the lentils and the water to the onions and bring to a boil.

Lower the heat, then add the bulgur to the pot, mixing it into the lentils and onions. Cover, and let it all simmer for 15 minutes.

When the water is almost gone, uncover and let it dry out a little over low heat.

Enjoy it with side salad or some vegan yogurt.

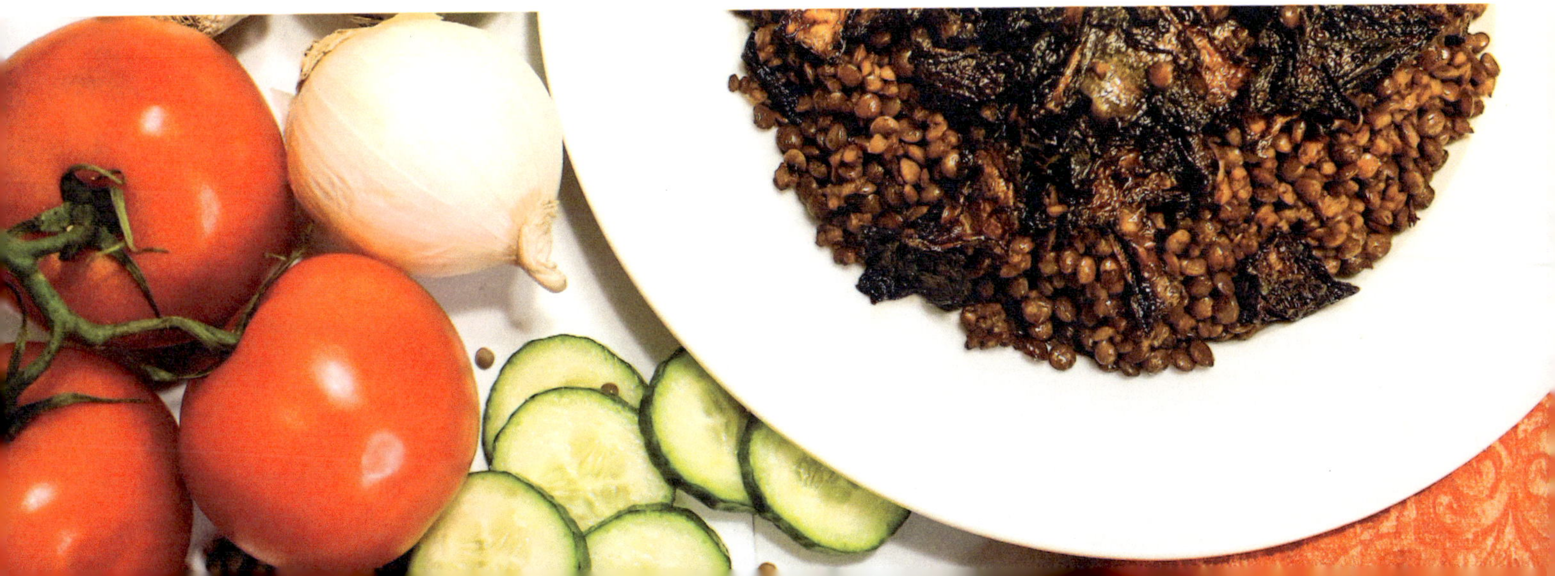

We all know people who have died from cancer. One of my father's employees, a good friend, died from it. We all know various cancers can be prevented, and that if we reached the moon, then we discover a cure for it. But since we cannot, we should focus on preventing what we can in our own bodies, right? Develop a healthy lifestyle, beginning with your diet, and changing your eating habits. Various studies have shown that even moderate increases in consuming plants lower our risks for multiple diseases,[7] but research from 2012 found vegans have lower overall rates of cancer than both meat-eaters and vegetarians.[8] We can't cure cancer yet, but we can do a better job of stopping it taking hold of us if we eat better and get some exercise.

We can't cure cancer yet, but we can do a better job of stopping it taking hold of us if we eat better and get some exercise.

Later Evening

I drink tea (herbal types) almost every evening, which is usually my time to sit, reflect and read more about (about health and veganism, but as you can tell from this book, it's not just my lifestyle, it's a massive part of who I am). I lived with teta most of my life. She would visit us for months at a time, and we would visit her. We were very close. We were best friends.

Yes, she and my mother taught me to cook, but she also taught me loyalty. As I mentioned earlier, she was only 27 when her husband died. She used to tell me, "I will meet with him when I die," and she would talk about him almost every day, even on her death bed.

As she grew older, I would help her. I found taking care of "my old lady" was easy and fun for me, and I would help her with things like manicures, dying her hair, showering, and also around the house. And, of course, we would bake and cook while we danced and sang.

Yes, she was my teta, but she was also my baby, and she's forever in my heart.

I would make juices and such when she needed something. If she was sick, I would make her *Magical Tea* (it's not really magic, of course, but it's what I think is the best herbal Turkish tea to treat the flu or a cold).

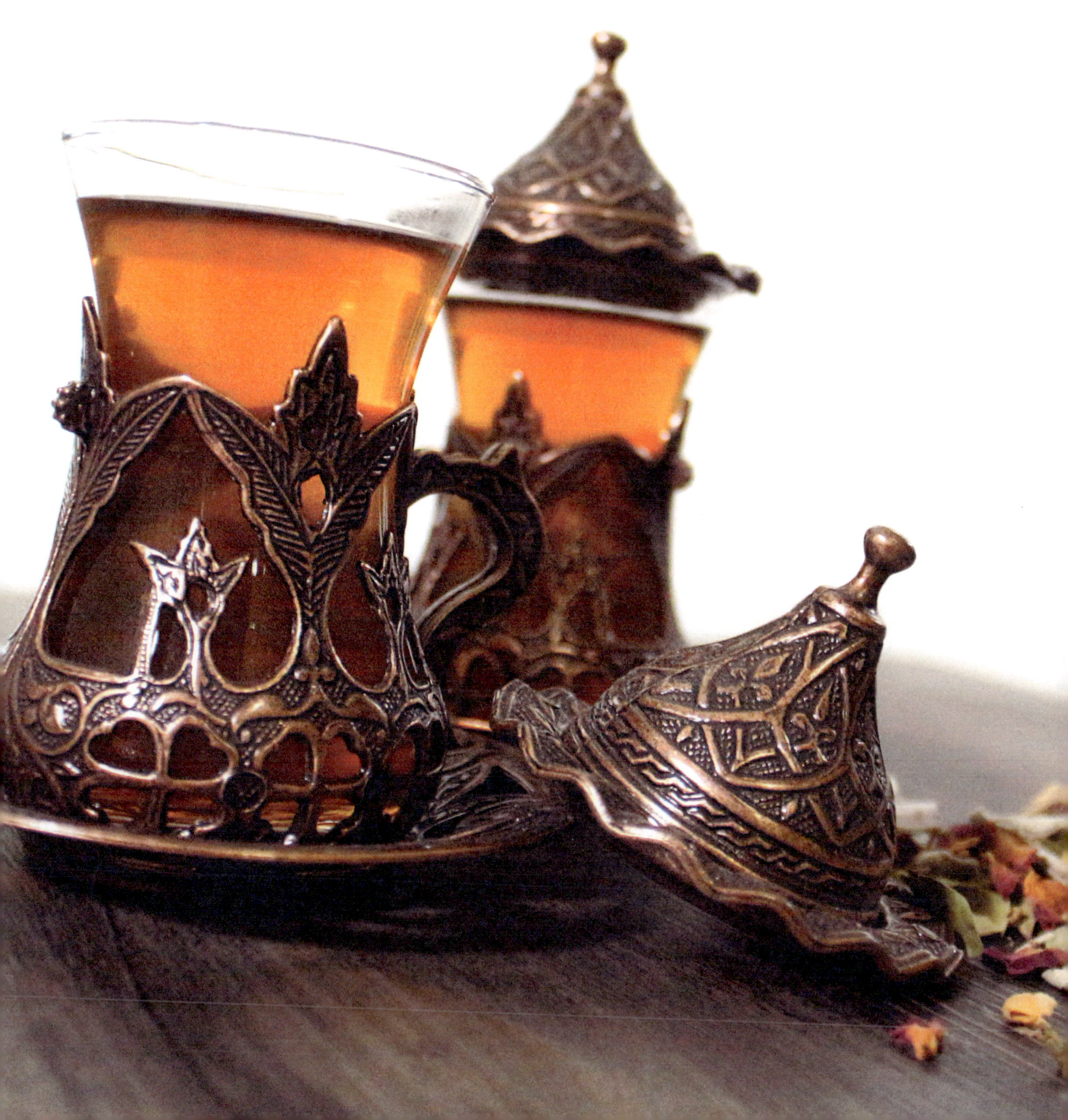

MAGICAL TEA

- Dried rose petals
- Linden flowers
- Sage
- Cinnamon stick
- Dried Oregano leaves
- Dried mint leaves
- Fennel seeds
- Licorice root
- Lemon balm
- Chamomile
- Chicory root
- Water

This will take some trial and error—just choose the amounts you think you would like! If it didn't suit you this time, adjust it for the next one.

Once you know what you want to use, put the herbs in a cup, bring the water to a boil, and then add the water to the cup just after the water comes off the boil (the rolling stops) and set aside to steep for 10 minutes.

Strain it if you like, and add a sweetener of your choice (or not—I don't use sugar in my tea).

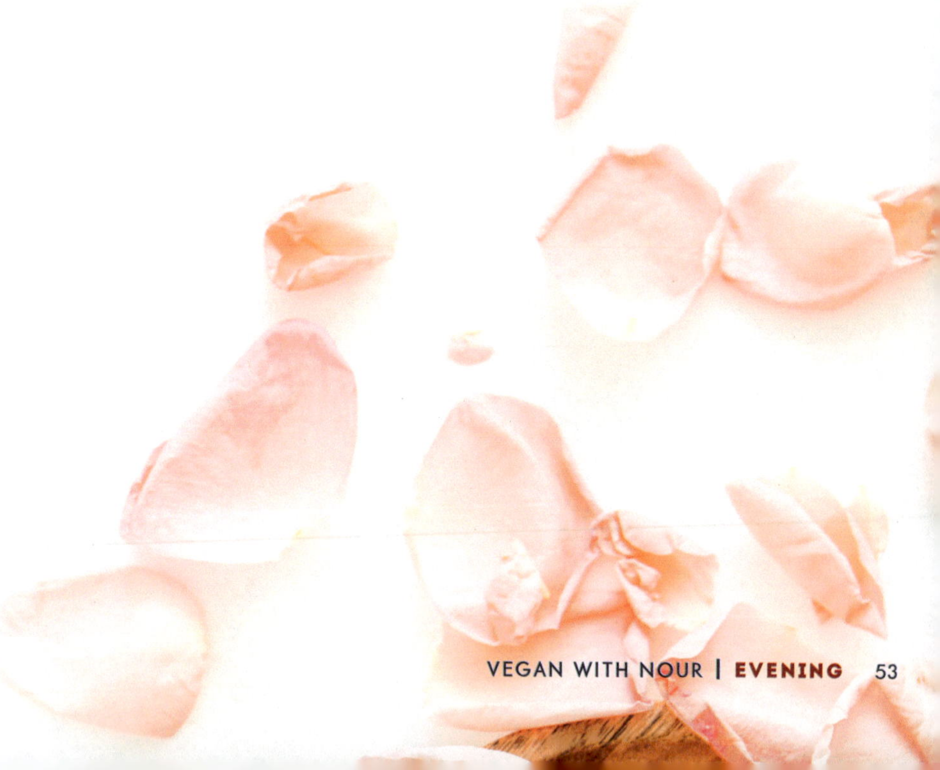

Menopause and veganism

Thinking of evening, and reflection, and how we age as women, the question of what happens after our child-bearing years is one of those questions that I'm asked by my older clients (though even if you are a teenager, it's essential you understand this, too—reflection is a good time to think about what the future holds for you).

My mother would say, "due to the influence of hormones, I could burst into tears or kill you in the next five minutes" when she was dealing with menopause. And it affects different women in different ways, such as:

- Irregular periods (until they end entirely)
- Vaginal dryness
- Hot flashes
- Chills
- Night sweats
- Sleep problems
- Mood changes
- Weight gain and slowed metabolism
- Thinning hair and dry skin
- Loss of breast fullness

I have helped relatives and clients with my home treatments to help remedy the effects. Hormone replacement therapies can carry a cancer risk with them,[9] and that's one reason why many doctors recommend avoiding those therapies (when possible). So what are we to do when dealing with a changing body as we age?

My mother, aside from casually informing me she might kill me or break into tears at any moment, would sweat in the middle of a cold winter (while Lebanon doesn't get as cold as the northern United States, it can get quite chilly). She'd ask me to open the windows and turn on the air conditioning… in winter. The hot flashes made her skin sticky with sweat, almost as if she was exercising on the beach in August!

The earlier you make these foods staples in your menopause diet, the more comfortable menopause

And, of course, when hormone levels change, they change everywhere across your body. During menopause, there will be points your body won't produce enough estrogen. And then, too much is produced. Your body tries to compensate, resulting in fatigue and memory loss.

I don't believe medicine can "cure" menopause (not that there's any way to cure something that is a natural part of our lives). The natural and organic ways are always my first choice for this.

Now, if those don't work, then you need to talk with your doctor. I can help, though, by showing you how going vegan can help with menopause.

Of course, many women have heard of the supplements and food we should consume before and after we reach menopause—and much of it is plant-based or easily substituted with plant-based ingredients. The earlier you make these foods staples in your menopause diet, the more comfortable menopause, and the years beyond, may be. It's never too late to go vegan.

Menopause and Exercise

I'm not going into exercise much in this book (see my blog at *VeganWithNour.com* for more about exercise and fitness), but it's important to point out that in menopause, like pregnancy and even just the regular parts of our lives, eating healthy and exercise are twins that should never be separated!

At one point, my teta (who did have osteoporosis) fell and broke her hip. I remember the doctor telling her if she had exercised more when she had been younger, there would have been less of a chance of that happening. Exercise is essential for menopausal and post-menopausal women, as it reduces your risk of disease, helps prevent weight gain (of course), and it can strengthen your bones after you complete menopause.[10] Life expectancy in America is on the rise again,[11] and if we're going to live longer, wouldn't it be nice to be as healthy as possible so we can enjoy it?

Exercise, a plant-based diet, and an overall vegan lifestyle will help!

Trust me, nothing will benefit your health and increase your chance of not dying as much as eating a plant-based diet. Go vegan for your health, your family and loved ones, the environment, and the animals. It's never too late—just do it!

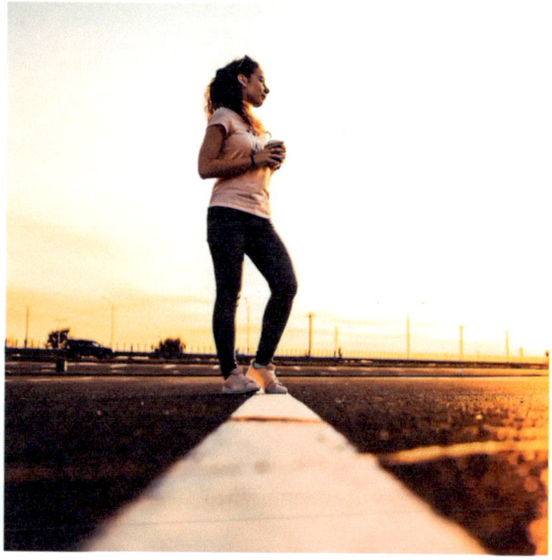

Let's start with the basics your body needs, especially before menopause:

- **Drink more water.** You probably already don't drink enough (upwards of 75% of American adults are chronically dehydrated[12]), and when we reach menopause and its decrease in estrogen, we can experience vaginal dryness, dry skin, and so on. Being properly hydrated (at least eight glasses a day, but find an online calculator to help determine the best amount for you) can help maintain your skin's moisture.

- **Get enough vitamin D.** Many of us have been marketed to about the importance of getting enough vitamin D before and after menopause. I discuss how vital vitamin D is for all of us in the Introduction. It's essential to understand it can protect your bones during menopause. Yes, vitamin D is created in the body from our exposure to sunlight, women's health needs usually mean taking a supplement to make sure you're getting enough (especially in winter and/or in non-sunny climates).

- **Focus on your calcium intake.** Estrogen loss can speed up bone loss, which means calcium will help. Fortified unsweetened soya, calcium-set tofu, rice and oat drinks, sesame seeds and tahini, calcium-enriched bread, and dried fruit (raisins, prunes, figs, etc.) all have calcium. There are also supplements you can take.

- **Consume more fruit and vegetables, especially ones low in calories.** This will help you avoid gaining weight as your metabolism slows down.

- **Watch your iron intake.** At the start, you may still need to boost it, but your iron needs decrease during menopause,[13] so talk to your doctor before making any changes to your iron intake or trying to increase it—you simply may not need it.

- **Eat more soy.** Soy compounds, called isoflavones, can mimic (not replace) estrogen in the body. Try to eat edamame, tofu, and other non-processed soy foods (stay away from the soy burgers for now) as much as possible. This should help curb your hot flashes.

» **Whole grains will help keep the digestive system functioning.** Some, such as steel-cut oatmeal, quinoa, barley, and brown rice, supply vitamin B, which helps boost energy.

» **Folic acid and fiber,** also found in whole grains, help lower risk for cardiovascular disease, which rises after menopause.

» **Lastly, I would say, eat more flax.** These are lovely seeds with omega-3 fatty acids, rich in fiber, and also provide phytoestrogens.

» **An excellent example of a recipe for easing menopausal symptoms,** partially due to its superb vitamin B6 content, would be my teta's beautiful and tasty *Bulgur and Tomato Kibbeh*.

In addition to what you should consume, what about what you should avoid?

» **Alcohol.** A drink a day won't worsen things, but there are increased risks of cancer and bone and organ damage.[14] Beyond that, research has found alcohol can make menopause symptoms worse,[15] so that "drink a day" might be best kept to a drink a week or less.

» **Sugar.** You want to avoid high blood sugar and insulin resistance, so keep your sugar intake low.[16] Yes, you can still have a reasonably-sized cookie, but switch to snacking on fruits (especially berries).

» **Caffeine.** It can make you even more tired,[17] especially if you drink it in the afternoon. If you're used to drinking coffee, keep the caffeine intake to 400mg or less per day (and reduce the sugar and creamer to reduce calories).

» **Root vegetables and spicy and warm foods** can raise your body temperature.[18] If you're already dealing with hot flashes, raising your body temperature isn't going to be fun. Avoid them (even if you love them).

» **And, aside from food, avoid tobacco.** Smoking has a direct connection to lower bone density,[19] and if you add that to everything your body deals with during menopause, it's best to quit.

» **I suggest veganism before, or even after, you reach menopause.** If you are younger and have older relatives or friends going through this, share some of the tips from here. According to my own research, conversations I have had, and various research studies,[20] it seems that vegan women experience no (or hardly any) menopausal symptoms.

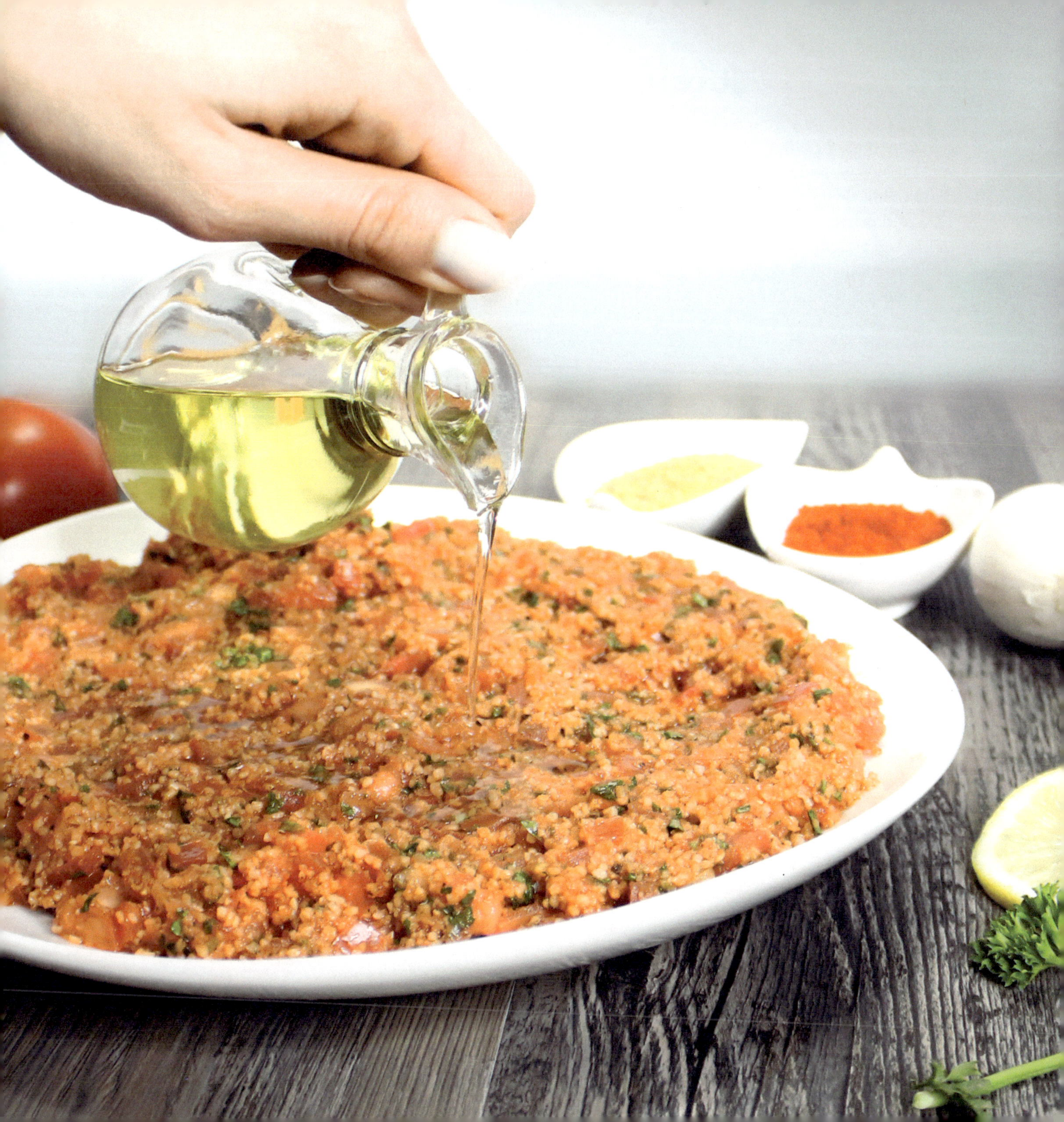

BULGUR AND TOMATO KIBBEH

2 big tomatoes
1 tablespoon of mint leaves
1 onion thinly chopped
1 red pepper
½ cup walnut
1 teaspoon black pepper
1 teaspoon cinnamon
1 tablespoon of dried red rose petals
¼ cup of dry basil
1 teaspoon cumin
A pinch of kosher salt
¼ cup of your choice of dry herbs (rosemary, sage, thyme, oregano, and others)
½ cup soft bulgur

Peel the tomatoes and cut them into a few pieces each, chop the mint leaves, slice the onion thinly, and cut the red pepper into a few pieces. Place that into your food processor bowl, then add the walnuts, black pepper, cinnamon, rose petals, basil, cumin, salt, and any other herbs you like. Mix it very well, breaking-down all the large pieces, turning it all into a paste.

Add the bulgur to the paste and then process it all for two minutes.

Serve with a side salad.

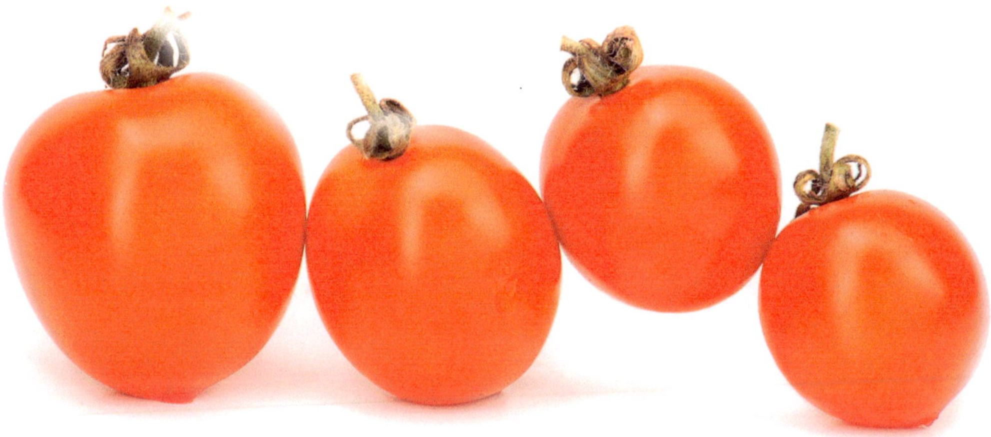

DOLMA

1 cup of rice
Water (I can't give any exact measurements here, but it will be a lot)
Ice (enough to help shock the grape leaves and onions)
2 large onions
2 large bell peppers
2 small eggplants
2 medium zucchinis
20 fresh grape leaves (up to 50 if you're not stuffing vegetables)
3 tomatoes
1 sprig of parsley
1 cup of mushrooms
5 cloves of garlic
1 red pepper
1 bunch of fresh dill
1 large red onion
1 cup and 1 tablespoon of olive oil
1 can of tomato paste
1 tablespoon of allspice
1 teaspoon cayenne pepper
Salt (to taste)
1½ cup of lemon juice

Just a note: Most Americans think of this dish as just stuffed grape leaves—but there is so much more to it! Dolma (literally meaning "stuffed") seems to be a traditionally Turkish dish that spread across Greece, the Middle East, Arabia, and is eaten by all of the peoples in those areas and in many different ways, and by all three of the major religions of the area. It's clearly popular! You can even stuff fruit (like quinces stuffed with rice, currant, and flavored with coriander, cinnamon, and sugar).

If want to do just stuffed grape leaves, then do so—it's great and tasty and you can easily increase the amount of grape leaves above to 30 or 40 for the amount of filling here. I like to do a mix of vegetables and grape leaves, so that's what I'm describing here.

Before you do anything, get a plate that fits into a large pot (it has to be something the vegetables can stand upright in and not stick out). Make sure you can push down on the plate easily and get it out easily, too. Then wash the bottom of the plate well (you're going to be pushing it against food) and set it aside (not on the bottom!).

Start cooking by soaking the rice. It should be ready by time you finish the prep work on the vegetables or leaves (and there's a lot to do):

DOLMA

Grape leaves can be delicate, so be careful with them (the rolling can forgive any small rips, but large ones are bad). Boil a pot of water and set a large bowl of ice water next to the stove. Blanch the leaves (not more than three minutes—you don't want them to lose their green color), and then quickly shock them in the ice water. Once they're cold, put them, as flat as possible, in a strainer to drain.

Hollowing out bell peppers is easy—slice the tops off and clear them out with just your fingers (make sure to get all the seeds and the white parts).

For eggplant, take off enough of the top to get inside and scoop out and create a deep bowl. Set the eggplant aside and keep the excess to roast and use in the *Eggplant Mutabbal Bowl* on page 45.

If you do zucchini, approach them like the eggplants—scoop out the centers and set them aside to use in something else.

Onions are difficult ones, but they're tasty! Peel the onions and boil them. Set up an ice water bath in a bowl that can hold all the onions. As soon as the onions are tender, fish them out from the boiling water and shock them in the ice water. Once cold, cut a slice off the bottom (where the roots were) to make the onion's bottom flat and it can stand on its own. Then cut a larger slice off the top (like a lid), and core the onions from the top, creating a bowl. Set the bowls and lids aside. You can save the bottoms and the insides for another recipe (such as the crispy onions for the *Kushari* on page 65).

Stuffing Directions

With all the veggies prepped, it's time to make the stuffing.

Drain the rice and put it in a large bowl.
Finely chop the tomatoes, parsley, mushrooms, garlic, red pepper, dill weed, and red onion. Add to the rice and mix.

Add 1 cup of olive oil, tomato paste, allspice, and cayenne to the rice and mix.

Add salt to taste. Mix one more time.

Now start stuffing the vegetables with the mix. When you get to the grape leaves, lay the leaf out with the points pointed away from you and the connection to the stem pointing toward you.

DOLMA

Put a dollop of the mix onto the leaf, fold the bottom pieces up, fold the sides in. Three sides are closed, one side (the top) is open, making it look like an open, leafy envelope. Roll (not too tightly) the portion with the filling away from you. You should now have what looks like a burrito made from a grape leaf. Don't worry if you get it wrong the first time—you'll get some practice in since you have about a dozen more to make!

Coat the bottom your pot with olive oil (some people will suggest layering the bottom with grape leaves—if you like that, go for it!), and arrange the dolma in the pot (the veggies need to be pointing with their openings upwards).

Pour the lemon juice into the pot (not into the veggies), then do the same with enough water to cover them with the plate on them (you might need to play with this a bit).

Press the plate firmly on the top of the veggies, cover the pot, and bring it all to a boil. Let it boil for five minutes, then reduce to a simmer for about 40.

Take a much-needed break, because the hard part is over. Once it's done, uncover, carefully remove the plate, and gaze upon your completed dolma!

Get a large serving platter and carefully take the dolma from the pot and arrange nicely on the platter.

If there is broth left, you can drain it from the pot and serve it alongside the platter.

Go sit down and enjoy!

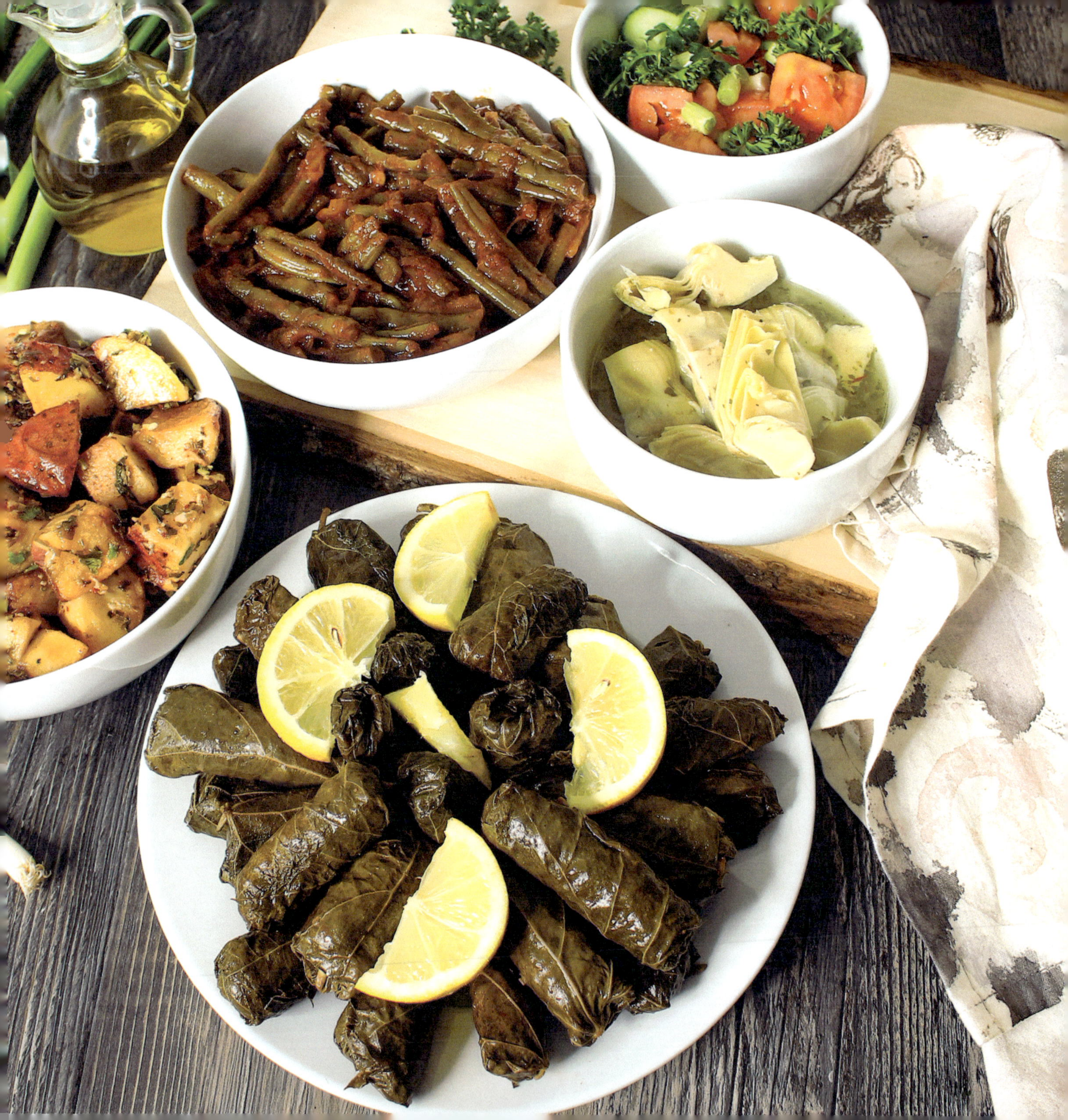

KUSHARI

This is one of the more complex recipes in the book, but I've broken it down into four steps to make it easier for you.

Onion Topping
1 large onion
A few pinches of salt
½ cup cooking oil
⅓ cup all-purpose flour

Tomato Sauce
1 small onion
4 cloves of garlic
1 tablespoon cooking oil
½ teaspoon of crushed red pepper flakes
1 teaspoon ground coriander
1 can of tomato sauce
A pinch of salt
2 tablespoons of white vinegar

Kushari
1½ cup of brown lentils
5-6 cups of water
¾ teaspoon and a pinch of salt (¼ teaspoon for lentils, ½ for lentils and rice, pinch for the pasta)
1½ cup of medium-grain rice
1 tablespoon cooking oil
½ teaspoon of pepper
½ teaspoon of coriander
2 cups of elbow pasta
1 tablespoon and a dash of cooking oil
Water
1 can chickpeas

Step 1 - Onion Topping
Slice the onion into thin rings and sprinkle them with salt.
Heat the cooking oil in a large skillet over medium-high heat. Create a landing spot (a plate with paper towel) for the onions to go after frying.
As the oil is heating up, coat the onions in flour, and shake the excess off.
Once the oil is ready, fry the rings, turning them often. Once they are a caramel brown (not burned), set them on the landing spot to cool.

Step 2 - Tomato Sauce
Grate the onion and mince the garlic, setting them aside in separate dishes.
Heat the oil in a saucepan over medium-high heat. Add the onion until the pieces turn translucent and start to turn golden (but don't let them brown). Add the garlic, red pepper flakes, and coriander and sauté for about 30, maybe 45 seconds, until it's fragrant. Remember to not overly brown the onions.
Stir the tomato sauce in along with the salt. Bring it all to a simmer and cook for 15 minutes or until it all thickens. Then stir in the vinegar, cover, and turn the heat to low. Leave it there until time to serve.

KUSHARI

Step 3 - Kushari
Clean and rinse the lentils (if you need to) and soak the rice while you cook the lentils.
Bring the lentils and the water to a boil in a medium pot over high heat. Once boiling, reduce the heat to low and cook for about 15 minutes (make sure the lentils are tender, but not fully cooked—you're looking for par-cooked). Drain them and season them with the salt.

Drain the rice from its soaking water and combine it with the lentils in the saucepan. Place it on medium-high heat, and add the cooking oil, salt, pepper, and coriander. Cook this for three minutes, stirring regularly. Add warm water (probably 3 cups or so) to cover the rice and lentil mixture by roughly 1½ inches. Bring it all to a boil, then reduce the heat to a simmer, and cover about 20 minutes (the rice and lentils need to be fully cooked and the water fully absorbed).

While the lentil and rice finish cooking, cook the elbow pasta (with the pinch of salt and dash of oil) until it is al dente. While the pasta cooks, put the chickpeas in a bowl, cover, and warm in the microwave for about 30 seconds. Then drain the pasta. Cut the crispy onion rings into 1-1½ inch pieces.

Step 4
To serve, bring it all together.
First, fluff the lentils and rice (use a fork, not a spoon), and place on a serving dish (a platter or a large plate). Top the rice and lentils with the pasta, half of the tomato sauce, the chickpeas, and half of the crispy onions. Place the remaining tomato sauce and onions for everyone to garnish as they see fit.
Serve.

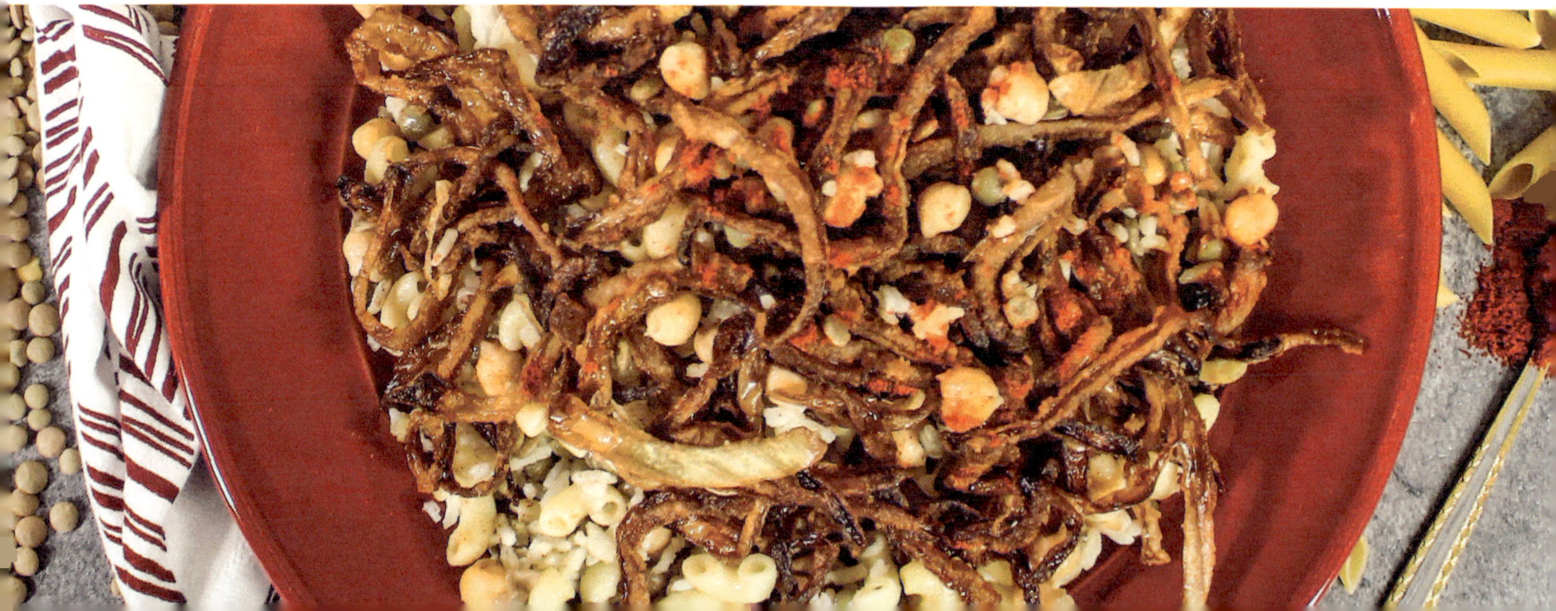

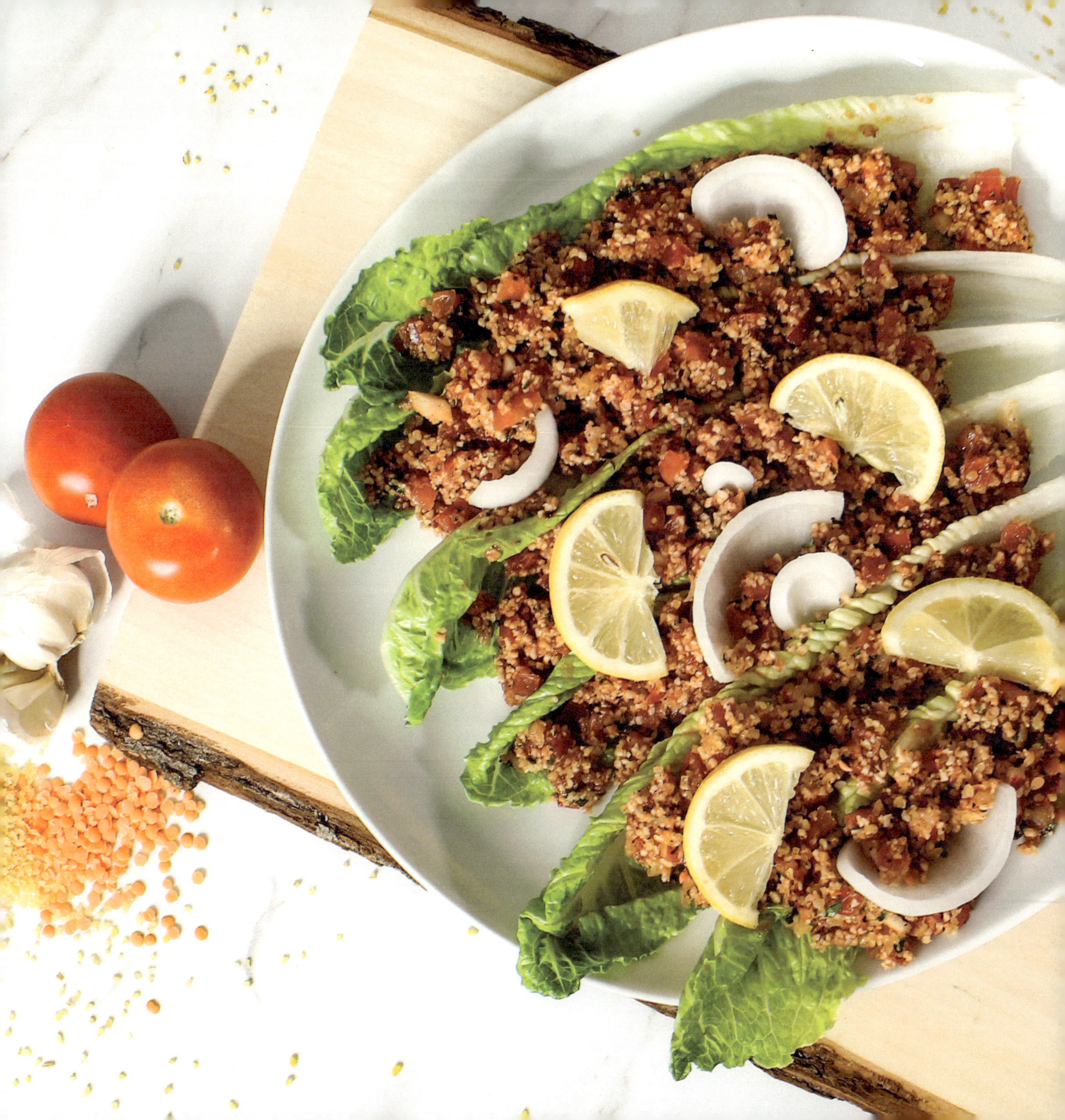

ÇIG KÖFTE

2 cups red lentils
3 large ripe tomatoes
2 cups fine bulgur
2 medium onions
5 cloves of garlic
1 tablespoon tomato paste
½ cup olive oil
1 tablespoon red pepper paste
1 teaspoon cumin
1 teaspoon salt
½ cup parsley
½ cup green onion
½ cup pomegranate molasses

Cook the red lentils by washing it and bringing it to a boil.

While the red lentils cook, peel and chop the tomatoes. Puree the tomatoes and set aside in a large mixing bowl.

Rinse the bulgur for few minutes in cold water. Drain them and add to the mixing bowl.

Drain the red lentils and add them to the mixing bowl. Add the tomato paste. Mix well, cover, and set it aside for about an hour (or until the bulgur is softened).

Roughly cut up the onions and peel and smash the garlic. Finely chop them up in the food processor, but don't puree them. Stir into the mixing bowl.

In a separate bowl, whisk together the oil, red pepper paste, cumin, salt. Add to the bulgur mixture along with the pomegranate molasses. Knead this all together, add salt if necessary, and then fold the parsley and green onion in.

Cover again and set aside for at least five hours (or preferably overnight).

When ready, put on food safe gloves and shape the çiğ köfte by putting 2 tablespoons of the mix in your hands and squeeze it with your fingers slightly separated. This creates a long stick shape with indentations from where your fingers compressed it.

Serve them on a bed of lettuce.

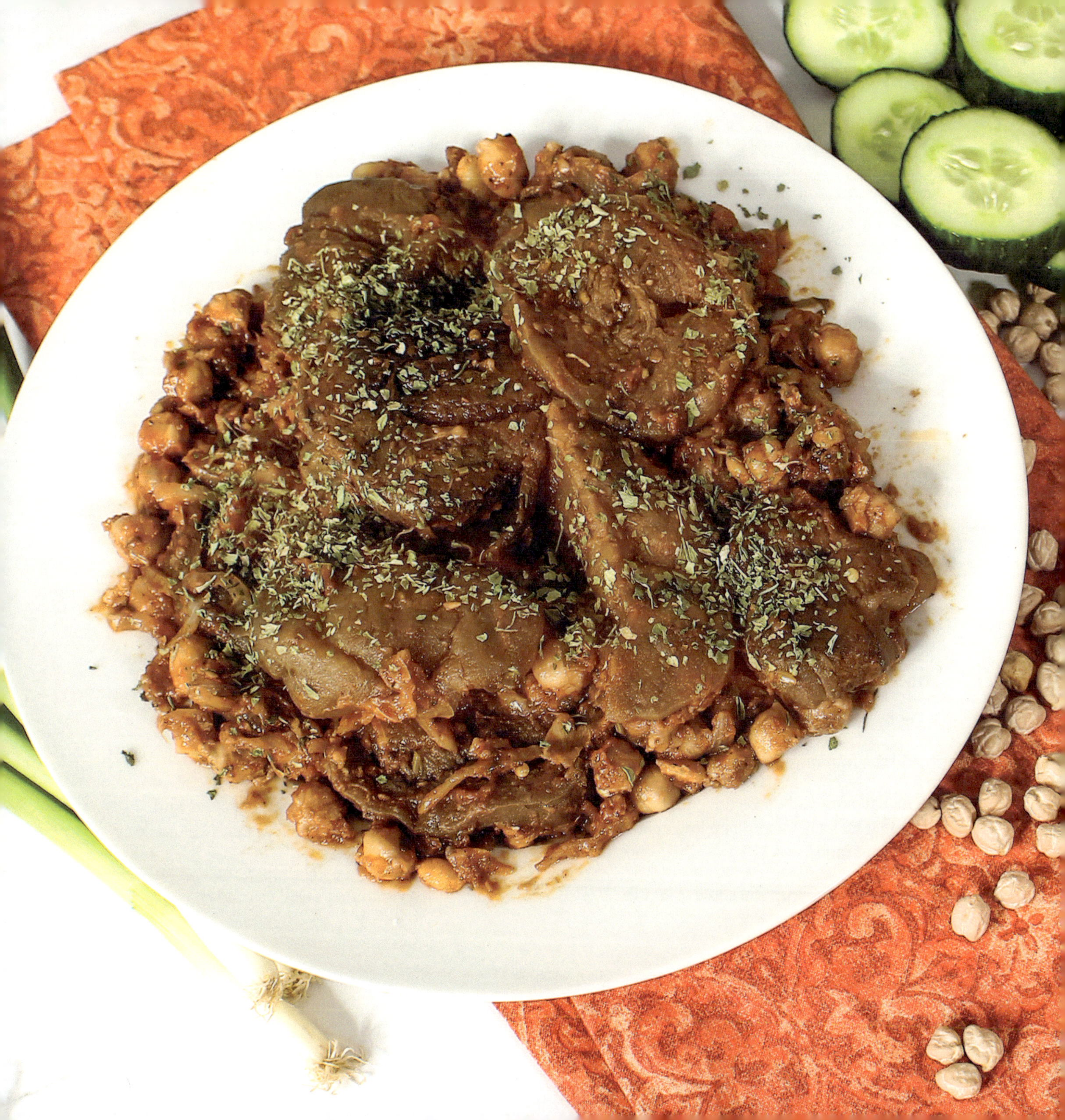

MAGHMOUR

1 large eggplant
½ cup of olive oil
2 medium onions
5 cloves of garlic
3 tomatoes
1 tablespoon tomato paste
1 can of chickpeas
1 tablespoon black pepper
1 tablespoon paprika
A pinch of kosher salt
¼ cup of dry mint (plus some to sprinkle over it when serving)

Preheat your oven to 400°F.

Peel and chop the eggplant (into medium-sized pieces), coat with half of the olive oil (¼ cup) and spread on a baking sheet until the oven is ready. Bake for 15 minutes.

Thinly chop the onions and set aside.

Peel and crush the garlic and set aside.

Peel and chop the tomatoes and set aside.

Heat the remainder of the oil (¼ cup) in a medium-sized pot. Add the onions and garlic, cooking until the onions are golden (not caramelized).

Drain the chickpeas and let them cook with the onion and garlic for a few minutes.

Add the tomatoes and tomato paste and bring it to a boil.

The eggplant should be done baking at this point, so add those pieces to mixture on the stove and bring it all back to a boil on low heat. Add the black pepper, paprika, kosher salt, and mint. Let cook just a bit more.

When serving, sprinkle some mint over it (I also enjoy this with a cucumber salad as a side).

ENDNOTES

1. www.cambridge.org/core/journals/public-health-nutrition/article/is-cooking-at-home-associated-with-better-diet-quality-or-weightloss-intention/B2C8C168FFA377DD2880A217DB6AF26F
2. www.livestrong.com/article/36880-vegetable-sources-cholesterol/
3. www.theconversation.com/got-high-cholesterol-here-are-five-foods-to-eat-and-avoid-63941
4. www.healthline.com/nutrition/eggplant-benefits
5. www.healthline.com/nutrition/artichoke-benefits
6. www.healthline.com/health/diabetes/diabetes-rice
7. www.escardio.org/The-ESC/Press-Office/Press-releases/reassessing-the-benefits-of-plant-based-eating-pure
8. www.pubmed.ncbi.nlm.nih.gov/19279082-cancer-incidence-in-vegetarians-results-from-the-european-prospective-investigation-into-cancer-and-nutrition-epic-oxford/
9. www.cancer.org/cancer/cancer-causes/medical-treatments/menopausal-hormone-replacement-therapy-and-cancer-risk.html
10. www.mayoclinic.org/healthy-lifestyle/womens-health/in-depth/fitness-tips-for-menopause/art-20044602
11. www.cnn.com/2020/01/30/health/us-life-expectancy-drug-overdose-deaths-cdc-study/index.html
12. www.waterlogic.com/en-us/resources/human-hydration-are-we-drinking-enough/
13. www.ncbi.nlm.nih.gov/pmc/articles/PMC2821138/
14. www.healthline.com/health/menopause/alcohol#1
15. www.tandfonline.com/doi/abs/10.1080/03014460500421338
16. www.healthline.com/nutrition/menopause-diet#foods-to-avoid
17. www.healthline.com/health/food-nutrition/coffee-makes-me-tired#how-to-prevent-this
18. www.livestrong.com/article/483701-foods-to-increase-body-temperature/
19. www.bones.nih.gov/health-info/bone/osteoporosis/conditions-behaviors/bone-smoking
20. www.pubmed.ncbi.nlm.nih.gov/29704911-vegans-report-less-bothersome-vasomotor-and-physical-menopausal-symptoms-than-omnivores/

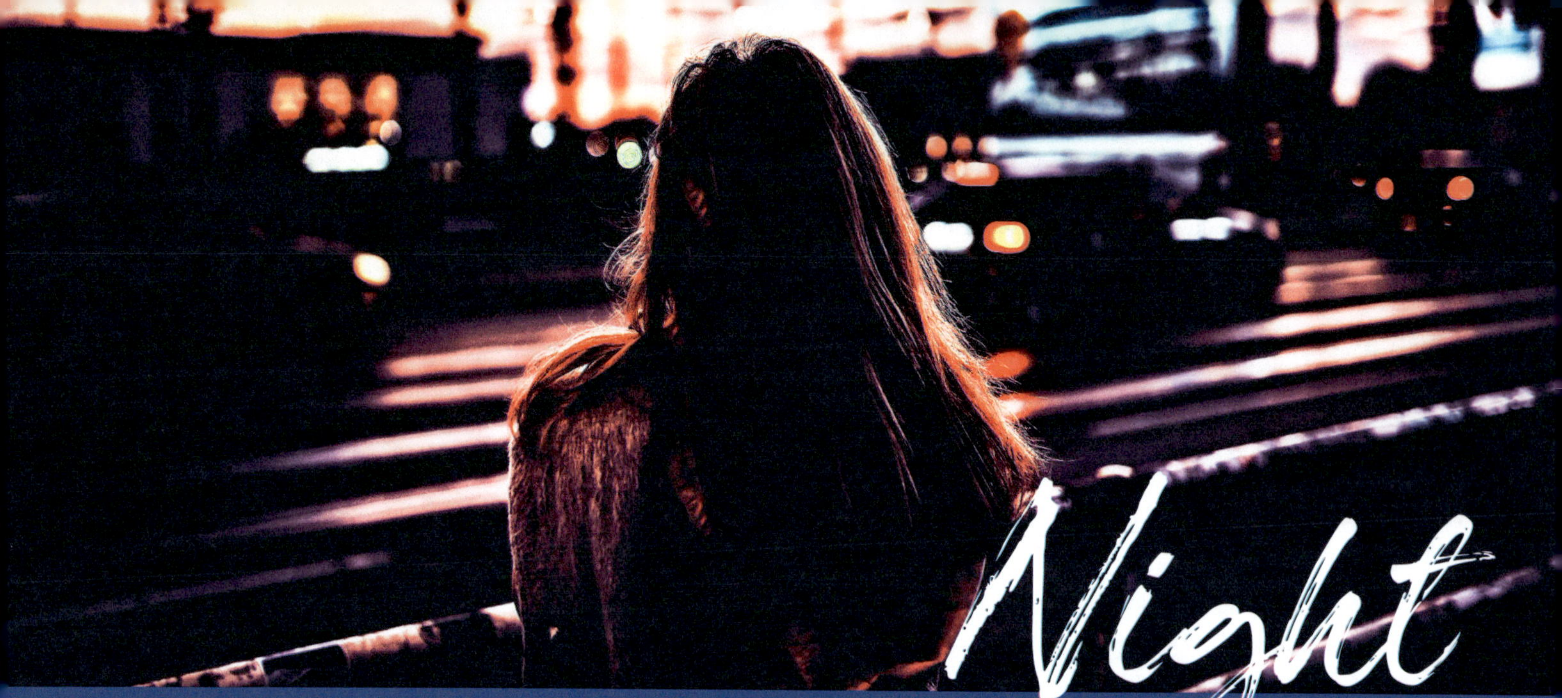

Night

Proper sleep and dreaming are cornerstones of a healthy mind, and those who take hold of their dreams and work will make them come true.

My childhood was full of fun, love, and wild events.

I remember running in fields, going on picnics, swimming in small lakes, and I clearly remember exploring old deserted houses.

One, built in 1753, must have been beautiful when it was new, with an ornate entrance, grand chandelier, and many windows throughout. What I really remember about it, though, is the old stairway to the basement. No, this isn't a horror story—there wasn't a monster waiting for us down there. But there was an old bathtub in the center of the room, ornate arches all around it. I asked teta later about that house and she told me a Turkish family had owned it, and what I saw was a Turkish bath ("hamam" in Turkish).

I have tried a hamam before. Now, Western art has shown it to be sexy and sensual, with a lot of nude women luxuriating around the room. It's not like that (regardless of how pretty those paintings might be). Usually women go to a hamam together (teta and I used to go together), but they wear towels around their bodies and sit in the hot air, scrub their bodies with an olive oil soap and loofah sponge, and then perhaps have a very rigorous massage. It's very healthy and relaxing. Of course, we can't all go to the hamam or the spa at the end of a long day, but isn't it nice to unwind in the bathtub after everything is settled for the day (with environmentally- and animal-friendly soaps and the like, that is)? Or, perhaps you like to unwind with a good meal and an indulgent dessert... but how indulgent can you be?

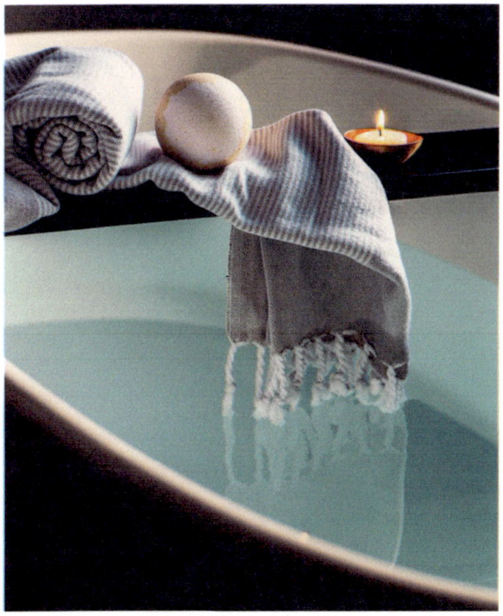

Desserts & Sleep

As it the day turns to night and bedtime comes closer, a vegan lifestyle still comes into play. Over the past decade, research into our need for good sleep as a society (and given a spotlight by Arianna Huffington's *The Sleep Revolution* in 2016) has become more and more frequent.

But how does being a vegan affect our sleep habits?

those who are overweight and eat more than 35% fat in their daily diet can double their severity of sleep apnea

One thing teta taught me when I was young is to not eat heavy at night. She would say "sleep light and you won't get nightmares," and what she meant was when you eat heavy before you go to bed you might end up experiencing insomnia because of the content of that food. And there is science to back her up.

A study has found that those who are overweight and eat more than 35% fat in their daily diet can double their severity of sleep apnea. The study goes on to note the severity also seems to increase when eating processed meats often or when more than two servings of dairy are consumed in a day.[1] Furthermore, an article on Bustle that discusses that study quotes a sleep expert who says because "Fatty foods are harder to digest, [they] can keep your body too busy to sleep. That means that fatty cuts of meat and high-fat dairy products, such as butter and cheese, can disrupt your sleep—especially if consumed in excess or the three hours before bedtime."[2] So, what's a good choice for a dessert at night before going to bed that's not going to destroy your sleep?

Meghli is a ground rice pudding that is topped with nuts. Starting when I was 10, I remember helping my mother in preparing this (it's one of my favorite Lebanese desserts), and not only is it vegan and very healthy, but it's so tasty! I would mix the ingredients and enjoy adding the toppings. Keeping with the pudding theme, the Turks have a pudding called *Ashure*, and it is traditionally vegan! It's said Noah made it of grains, fruit, dried fruit, and nuts (if you have an ark with *all* the surviving animals on it, would you eat any of them?). It's very tasty, and, again, you have all those great nuts and seeds in there.

I also love *Sfouf*! This is a turmeric, semolina, and almond cake. It is a cake, so maybe not eating it right before you go to bed is best, but it's not high in fat and it's very good. It can also last up to week unrefrigerated (not that I have ever seen it sit around for that long).

Different people make their desserts differently, so play with the recipes. One variation I've seen is to top things with walnuts. Remember how important B12 is? And that walnuts can pack a ton of B12 in a small serving? Well, there's evidence that lack of B12 (not just in pregnant ladies) and other vitamins can affect your sleep.[3] Put some walnuts on that meghli or sfouf (or just eat them plain)!

a lack of B12 and other vitamins can affect your sleep

Look, I won't lie—I snack at night also! I mean who doesn't like snacks, right? But I snack healthy so I can sleep well and guilt-free.

Late Night

I get it—you want to go out with your partner or your friends and have fun sometimes, but maybe that late night dessert of 20-layer chocolate cake with peanut butter mascarpone cheese and ice cream on the side (this is a real thing!) isn't such a wise choice (for your sleep, your waist, or the animals the cream, eggs, and milk came from)!

There is nothing wrong with going out for dinner and gatherings or grabbing something to eat after going dancing. There isn't even anything wrong with some alcohol, but try not to overdo it because it can hinder weight loss[4] and contribute to sleep issues, too[5] (no, getting drunk and passing out isn't considered "good sleep"[6]).

Wherever I go at night, my number one choice to eat is vegetables or fruit—you can usually find a way to order or pick something plant-based. Don't feel bad or mad that you aren't eating the same things the others are—this is for you! If one reason you have for going vegan is you want to get in shape and stay in shape, then you have to work on it.

Going vegan means not only treating animals and the Earth well, but treating your body well. You can kick back and enjoy yourself, but be reasonable. As we've seen throughout the book, if you invest in your body, and learn what it needs to serve you well—regardless of your stage in life—it will pay you back!

MEGHLI

2 cups of rice flour
6 cups water (2 cups to start, then the remaining later)
½ cup coconut sugar
1 teaspoon cinnamon
2 tablespoons caraway
Shredded coconut
Pistachios
Raisins
Pine nuts

Soak rice flour in 2 cups of water for two hours.

After the flour is done soaking, boil the remaining 4 cups of water in a large pot. While the water boils, prepare the sugar, cinnamon, and caraway and put them within reach of the stove.

Once the water boils, mix the soaked rice flour into the pot with a whisk. Keep the heat at medium and add the sugar and spices slowly—whisking constantly. Stir occasionally until it all thickens (about 50 minutes).

Pour into bowls, garnishing with the nuts, raisins, and shredded coconut.

Let them firm up and chill in the refrigerator for three hours, then serve.

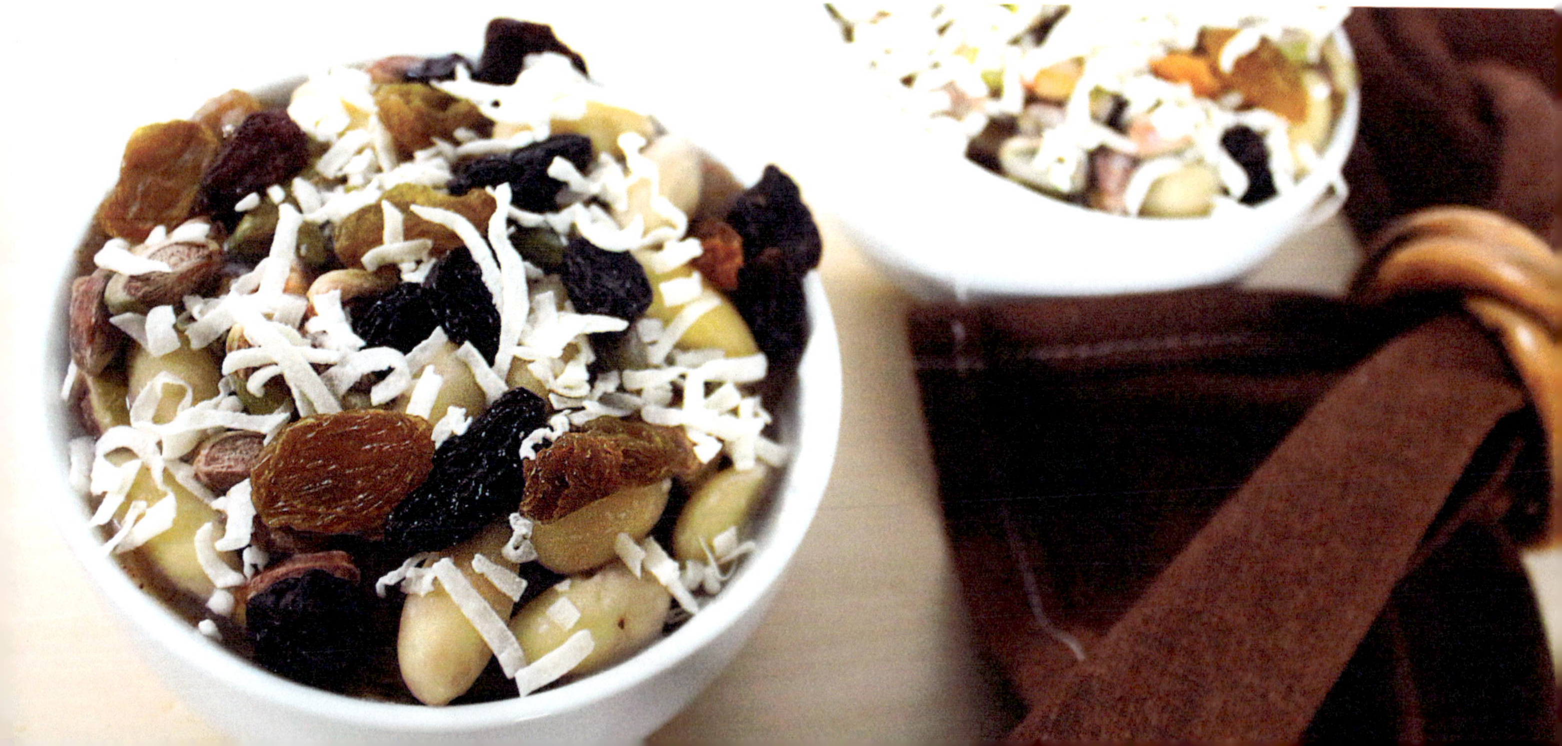

AŞHURE

½ cup barley
2 ounces of dried figs (optionally, also have some for garnish)
2 ounces of raisins
2 ounces of dried apricots
6 cups water
⅓ cup cooked or canned chickpeas
⅓ cup cooked or canned white beans
2 ounces peeled almonds
1 apple
1 teaspoon salt
1 cinnamon stick
½ cup almond milk
1 cup sugar (or honey)
Pomegranate seeds (optional)
Grated coconut (optional)
Blanched almonds (optional)
Roasted hazelnuts (optional)
Pistachio (optional)

This recipe takes prep work, so read it fully.

Start by soaking the barley overnight. When ready the next day, wash the figs and then boil for three minutes, drain them, and set aside. Repeat with the raisins—wash, boil for three minutes, drain, set aside. Wash the apricots and immerse them in water for 30 minutes. Drain the apricots, save the water you soaked them in, and then dice them.

In a large pot, cook the barley in six cups of water (or according to its package instructions). Add water if necessary. Cut the apple into large pieces (you will be removing them from the final dish). Halfway through cooking the barley, add the apple and the cinnamon stick and continue cooking until the barley is very tender—almost like porridge. Toward the end of cooking the barley, remove the apple and the cinnamon stick.

Then add the raisins, the apricots, and their soaking water to the barley, then put in the chickpeas, white beans, almonds, salt, sugar (or honey), and almond milk. Mix it all well and simmer for 10 minutes.

While simmering, dice the cooled figs. Mix the them into the barley at the end of cooking.

Transfer into pudding cups or ramekins and let it cool down. Top with more figs or any of the other optional garnishes. Serve at room temperature or refrigerate and serve cold.

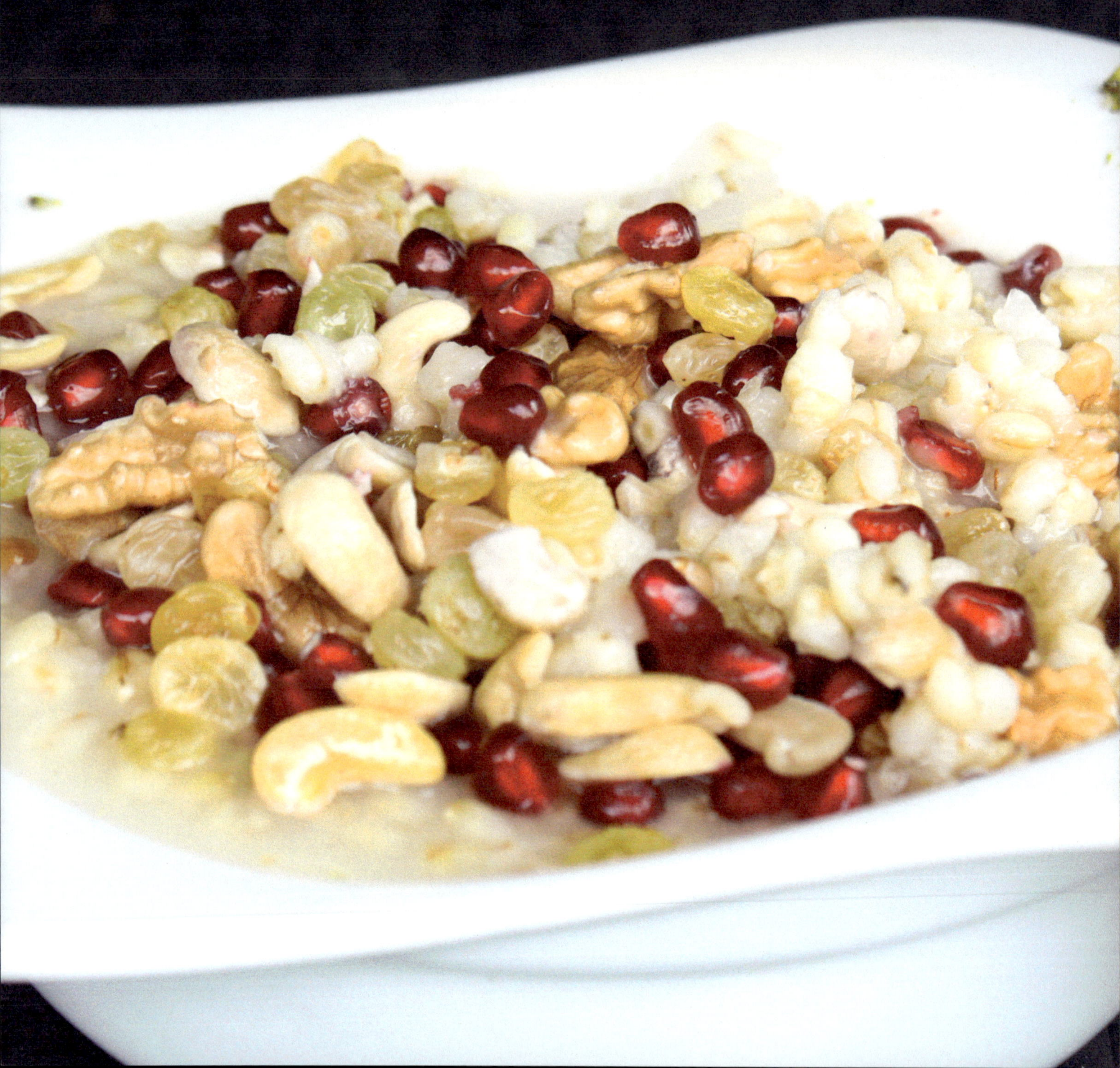

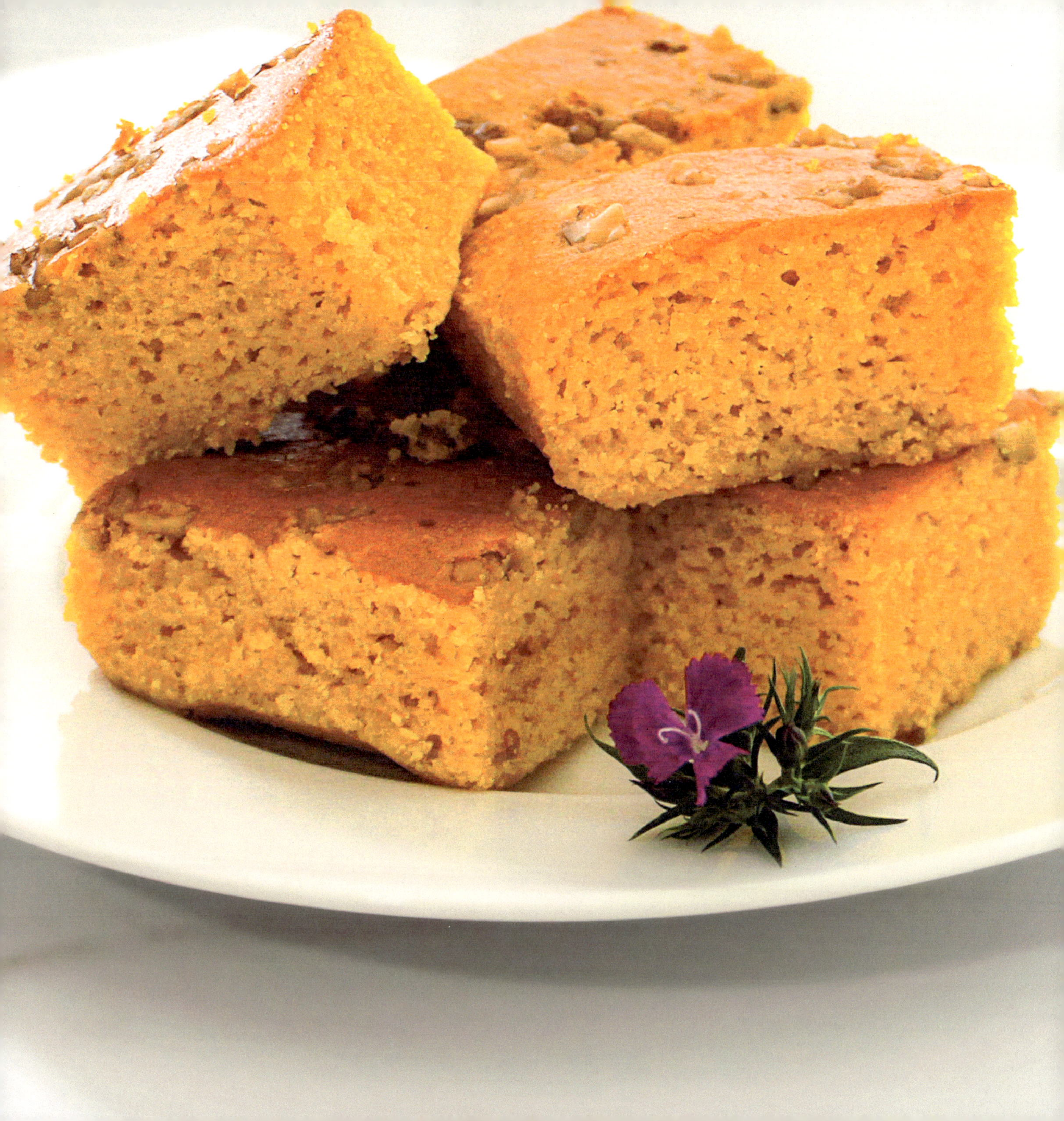

SFOUF

1½ cups semolina
1½ cups almond flour
1½ cups almond milk
3 teaspoons baking powder
1 tablespoon vanilla extract
1½ tablespoon turmeric
2 cups brown sugar
2 cups coconut oil
1 cup tahini
Approximately 2 cups of water
Slivered almonds

Preheat the oven to 375° F.

Mix the semolina, almond flour, almond milk, baking powder, vanilla extract, turmeric, brown sugar, coconut oil, and tahini together well. Add water until it's smooth and creamy, like vegan yogurt (and, if you don't need it all, don't use it; if you need more, add it slowly). Set aside.

Evenly spray cooking oil in an 8x10 or 8x8 pan. Spread the mixture evenly and sprinkle almonds across the top (how much is up to you).

Place the pan in the oven and bake for 40 minutes (use the toothpick test to make sure it's fully baked). Let it cool, then cut it into squares and serve.

It can last up to seven days in the refrigerator, but I've never seen it stick around that long.

BAKLAVA

½ cup of water
2 cups of sugar
1 tablespoon of lemon juice
20 sheets of phyllo dough (covered with wax paper and a damp towel to keep them moist)
2 cups of your favorite nuts, finely chopped
1 cup of your preferred vegan butter or margarine
Pistachios (optional)

If you decide to try making your own phyllo, go for it (it's not difficult) but making baklava with pre-made phyllo is just fine, too! Decide what works best for you. If you're making your own, give yourself enough time beforehand so the dough is ready.

Preheat the oven 350° F.

In a medium saucepan over medium heat, mix the water and sugar until it boils. Add the lemon juice and leave 15 minutes as the mixture becomes somewhat thick and heavy (don't let it burn), then remove it from the heat and let it cool.

Melt the vegan butter in the microwave so you can brush it.

Take baking pan, large enough to hold the full sheets of phyllo and with raised edges, and grease it with the vegan butter (or use parchment paper).

One at a time, remove a sheet of phyllo from the pile (remember to cover the others again), and grease it with the vegan butter using a brush. Repeat that process another nine times. Then take 2 cups of your favorite nuts and cover the top of the dough. Then repeat the process with the phyllo—take a sheet, lay it down, and brush it. Once you are done, you should have a 10-sheet layer of phyllo on the bottom, a layer of nuts in-between, and another 10-sheet layer of phyllo on top.

Unlike a lot of baked goods, you want to cut these before they go into the oven. My mother cuts them diagonally, creating diamond-shaped pieces, but you can do squares or rectangles. Just make them as even as you can.

Bake them for 15 minutes or until the top starts to turn a golden color.

Remove from the oven and pour the cold sugar syrup over the pieces, and (optionally) crush and sprinkle pistachios across the tops to decorate. Serve after the syrup has soaked into the pieces.

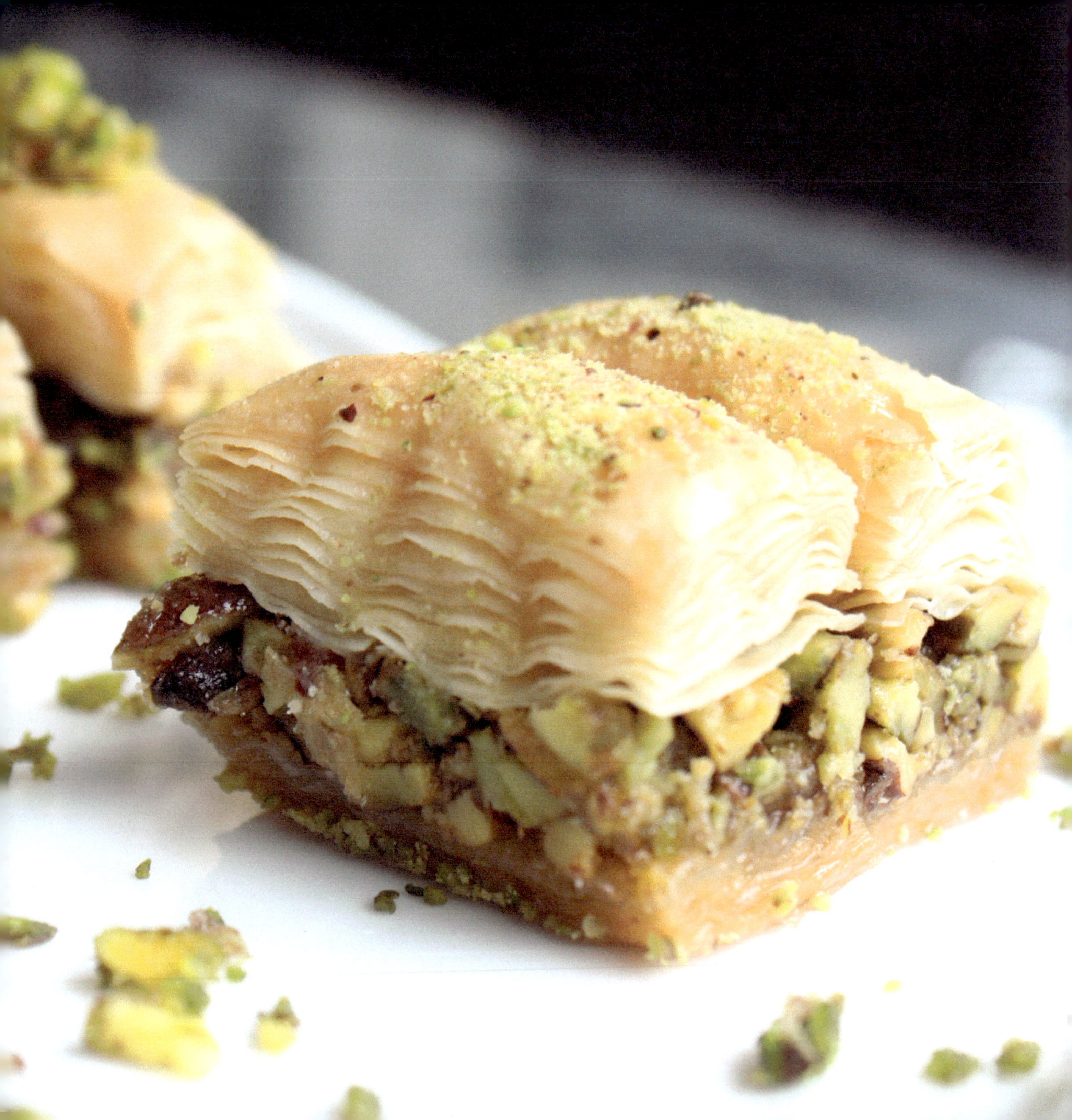

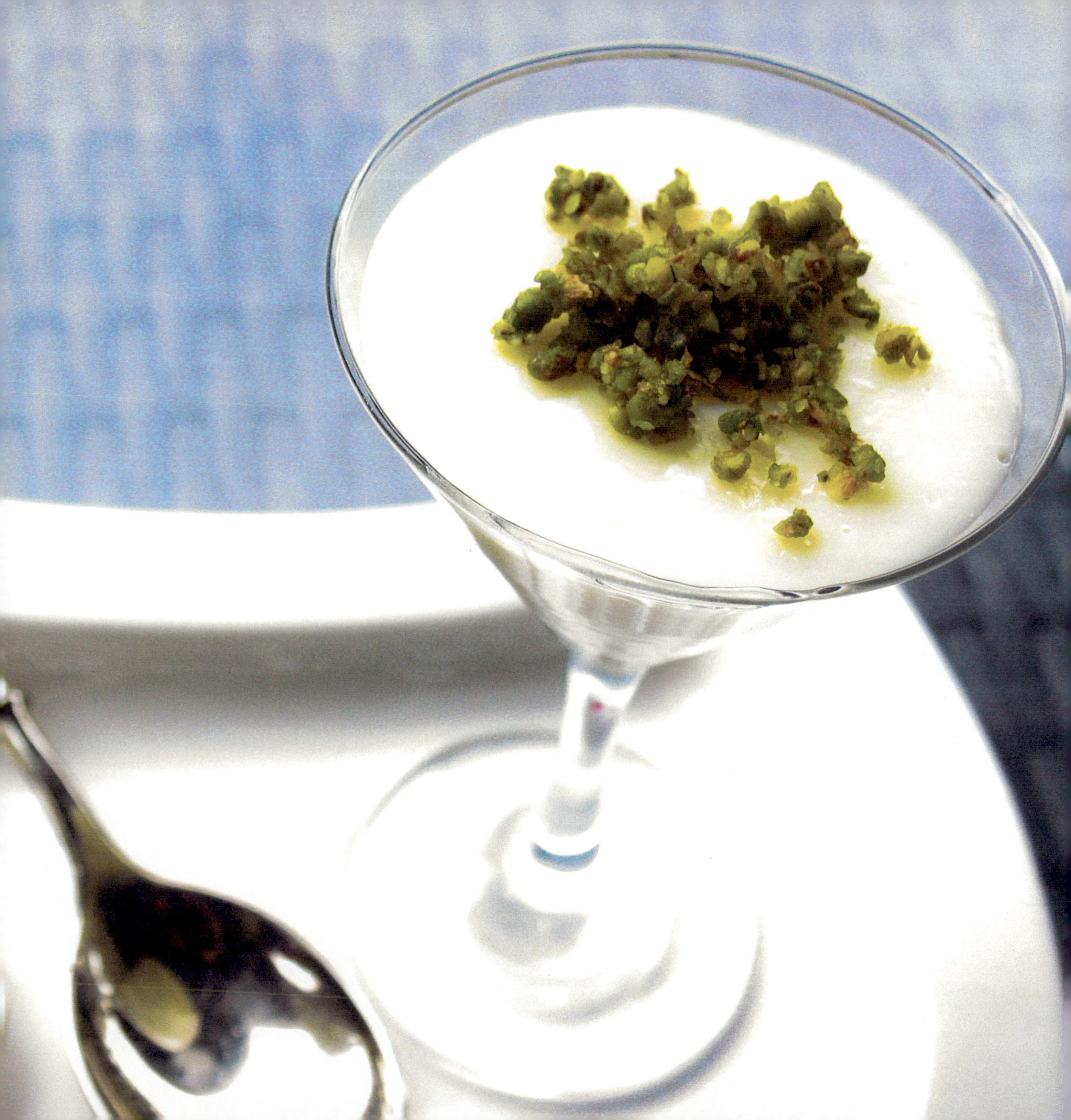

MUHALABEYA

4 cups of almond milk
5 ounces of sugar
5 tablespoons of cornstarch
1 tablespoon rose water
1 teaspoon of crushed cardamom
Agave or maple syrup
Crushed pistachios

In large saucepan, combine the almond milk, sugar, and cornstarch. Stir to mix them well and bring to a boil on medium heat, stirring occasionally

Once it starts getting thicker, lower the heat and keep stirring until it resembles a thick custard (make sure it doesn't burn!).

Once it's thick, take it off the heat and add the rose water and crushed cardamom and stir.

Pour into small bowls or pudding cups and let them cool down and set. Once they're no longer hot, place in the refrigerator to get cold (it will thicken more).

To serve, drizzle syrup over it and sprinkle with pistachios.

MADLOUKA

2 tablespoons vegan butter
⅓ cup semolina
4 cups of whipped coconut cream (2 in the madlouka, 2 for topping)
3 cups cashew or almond milk
1 cup sugar
2 cups of pistachios (crush or grind most of them, and leave some whole) for garnish

Melt the butter in a saucepan over medium heat.

Add in the semolina and 2 cups of the whipped cream. Then add in the cashew or almond milk and stir until it becomes thick.

Add the sugar and continue stirring until it forms a paste and remove the saucepan from the heat.

Mix well and let cool.

Once it's cool, spread it in a shallow serving dish, and top it with the remaining 2 cups of whipped cream, and sprinkle the ground pistachios (or cashews or almonds, if you prefer) and decorate with the whole ones before serving.

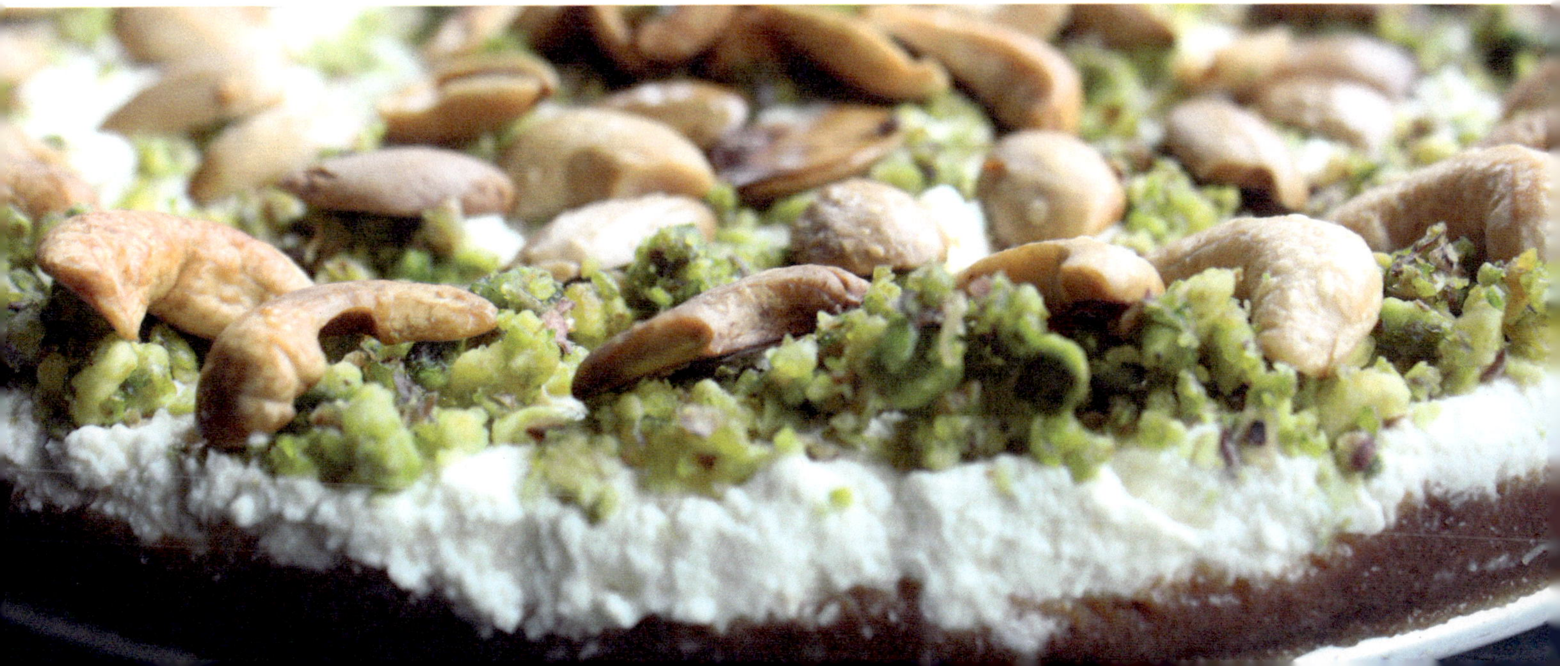

ENDNOTES

1. www.journals.sagepub.com/doi/abs/10.1177/1559827618765097
2. www.bustle.com/p/going-vegan-has-impact-on-your-sleep-a-new-study-shows-20511005
3. www.psychologytoday.com/gb/blog/sleep-newzzz/201905/5-ways-vitamin-deficiencies-can-impact-your-sleep
4. www.healthline.com/health/alcohol-and-weight-loss
5. www.psychologytoday.com/us/blog/sleep-newzzz/201801/alcohol-and-sleep-what-you-need-know
6. www.bustle.com/articles/154241-7-things-that-happen-to-your-body-when-you-go-to-sleep-drunk

CONCLUSION

It took me almost nine years to finish this book and I have enjoyed every minute of it! It's gone through many different versions, but I'm thrilled this is its final form! I hope you enjoyed it, and I hope it has made you think about how you can follow me on this journey!

Looking good to oneself, feeling good about oneself—this comes from within. We have to determine what "good" means for ourselves. Realistically, we can't work out and then eat fast food. To see good results, we should eat clean and take care of our bodies. In the introduction, I shared the benefits of going vegan and its positive effects on our health. I think the other chapters reinforce that, creating a framework you can build off of to help you to go vegan and get fit.

I know it's hard to change our lifestyle, but once you start, nothing can stop you. All I wrote is based on experience. When I was a teenager and had my miserable days, I hated to face the mirror. I had to justify my vegetarianism and fight family to not slaughter various animals. I shared a room with my sister and had to put a mat between our beds to work out, and there were days I didn't want to do that.

It's not easy, I know. But it's okay, always remember the beauty is what's inside—have peace with yourself inside and it will show through.

Don't wait till next week—start today! Go vegan and change your life! Not only are you no longer participating in animal suffering, you're actually learning new things! I studied nutrition in college, and, after going vegan, I learned many new things about veganism that I didn't learn in school. As you explore food and health, you learn about the ethics of animal suffering, and the incredible waste that comes from eating animals. You also get to try new recipes, learn about other ethnic cuisines, and possibly come across vegetables and grains you otherwise wouldn't (azduki, quinoa, and kale, to name a handful). Hopefully, by telling my stories and experiences, I've already exposed you to new ideas and foods, and you've become more and more glad that you want to make that change. I wish to be still alive when the whole world realizes the effects of using animal products and goes vegan.

If you want to know more about my exercise routines and more recipes, come to my website, *VeganWithNour.com*, and check out my blog and follow me on social media from there. If you have questions, feel free to drop me a line—I'd be more than happy to talk.

Remember, above all, you're beautiful.

You are beautiful.

Be yourself, make these changes for yourself, and be the beautiful person you are.

Thank you for reading!

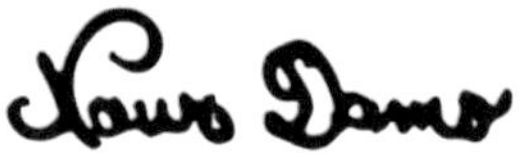

Nour

Be yourself, make these changes for yourself, and be the beautiful person you are.

RECIPE INDEX

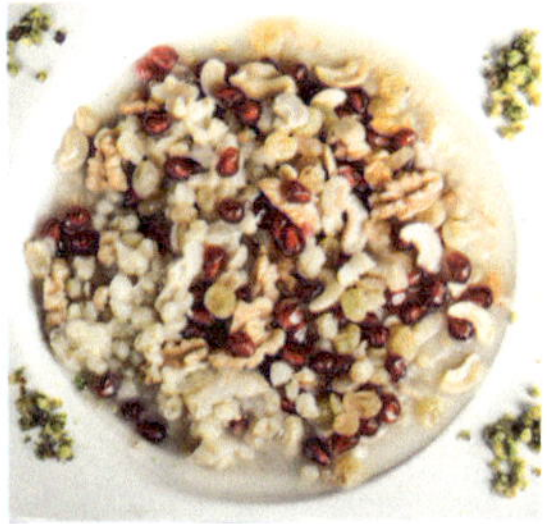

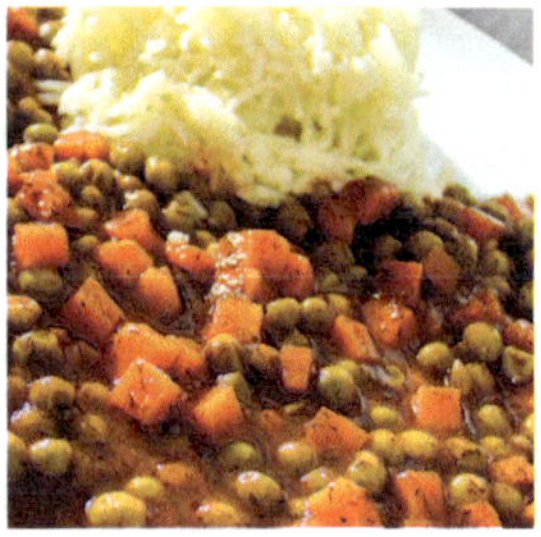

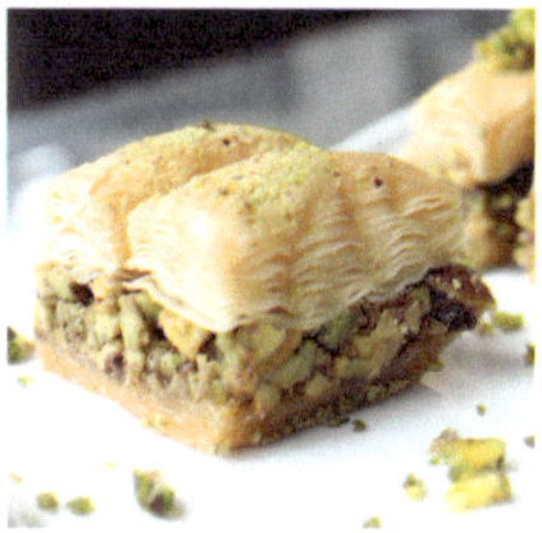

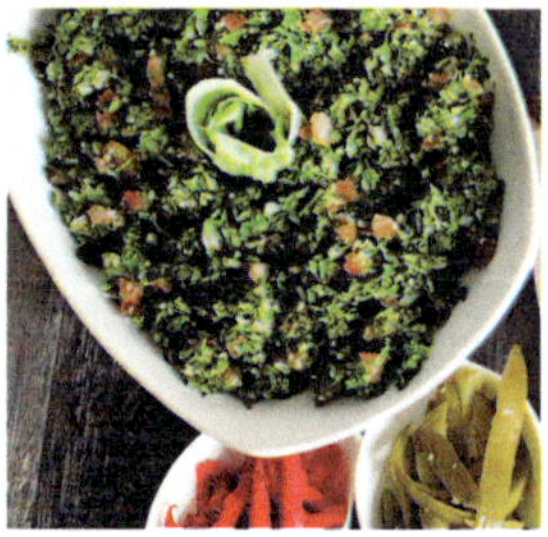

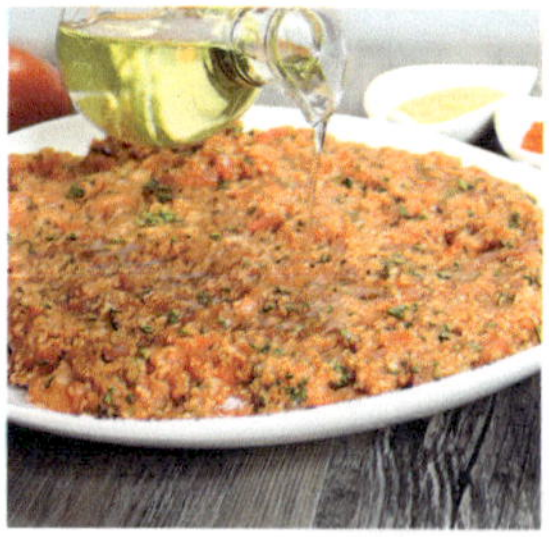

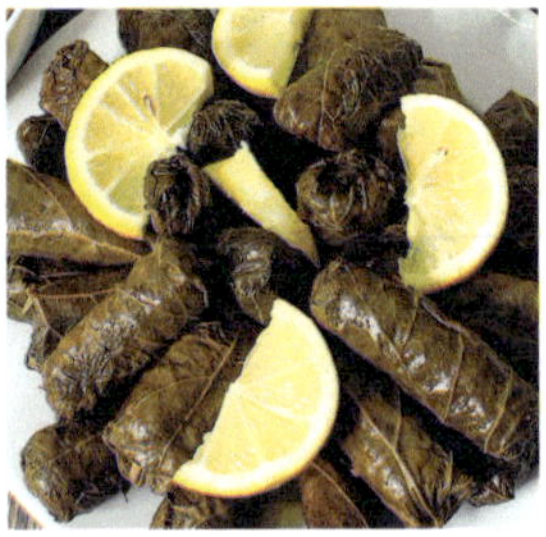

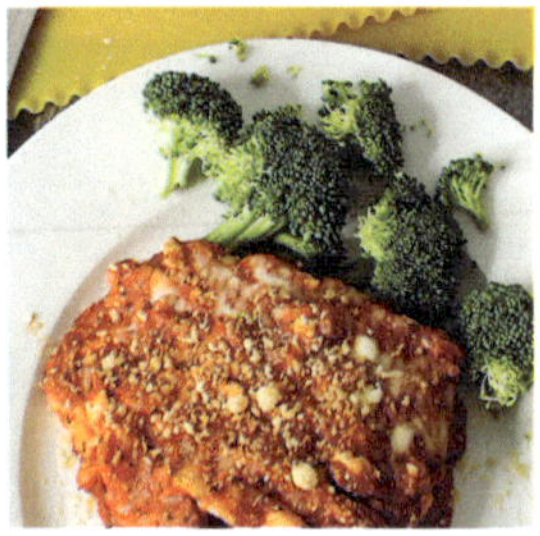

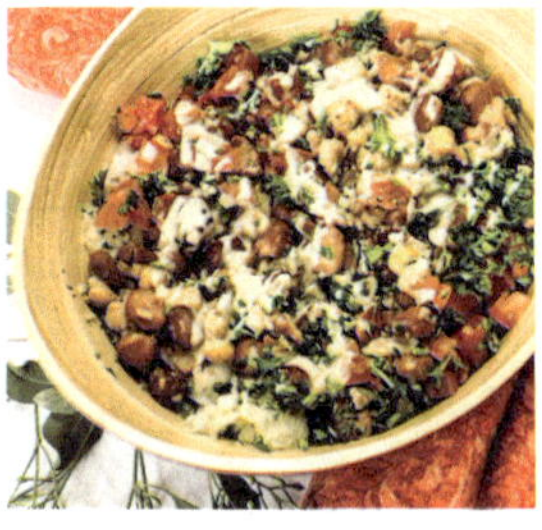

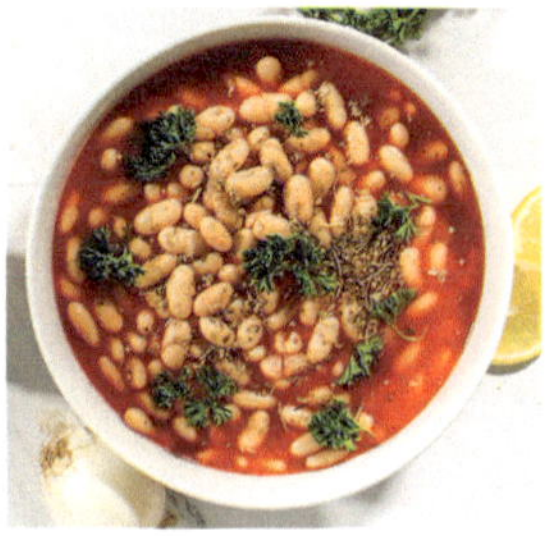

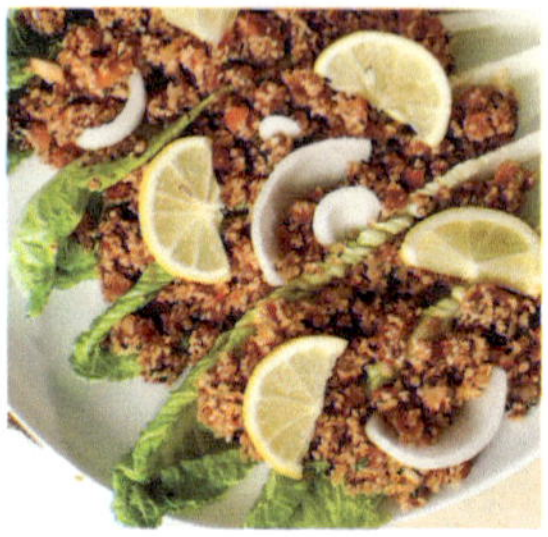

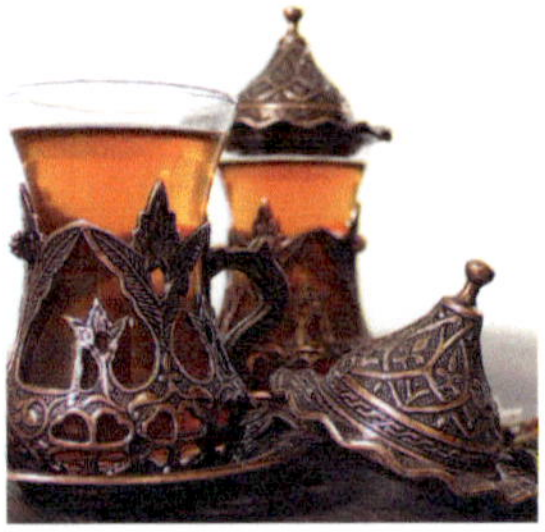

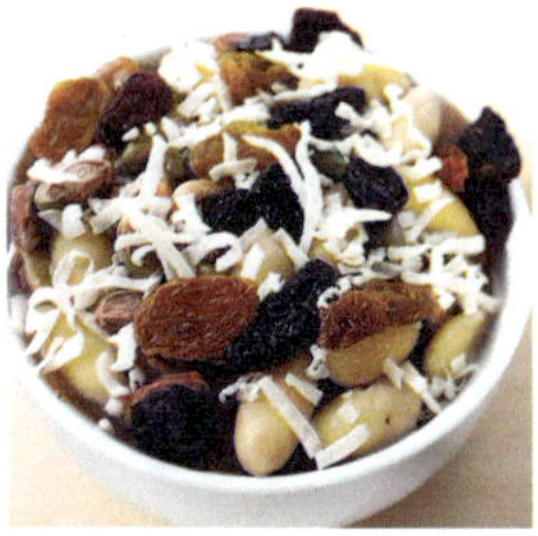

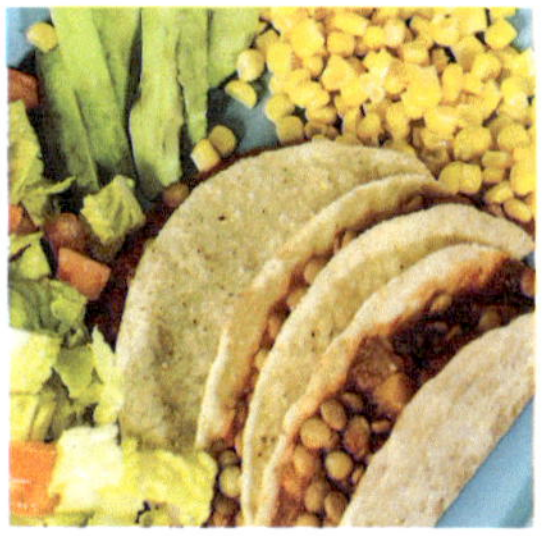

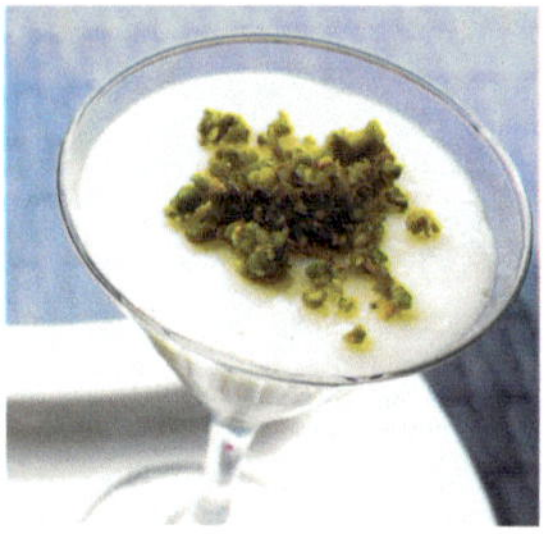

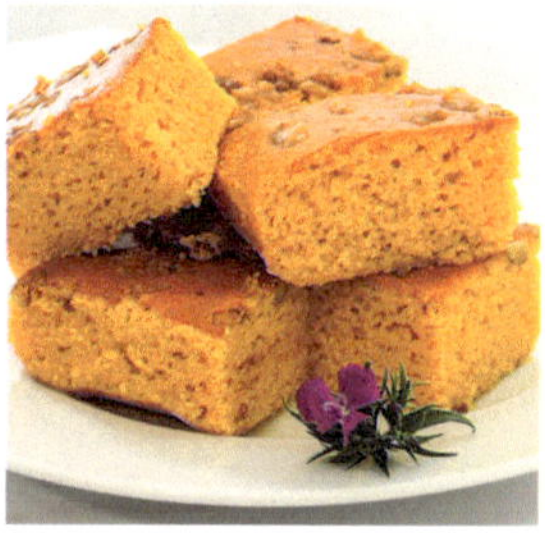

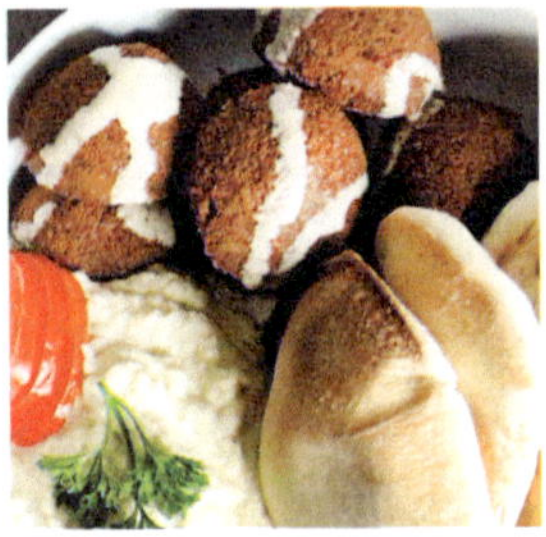

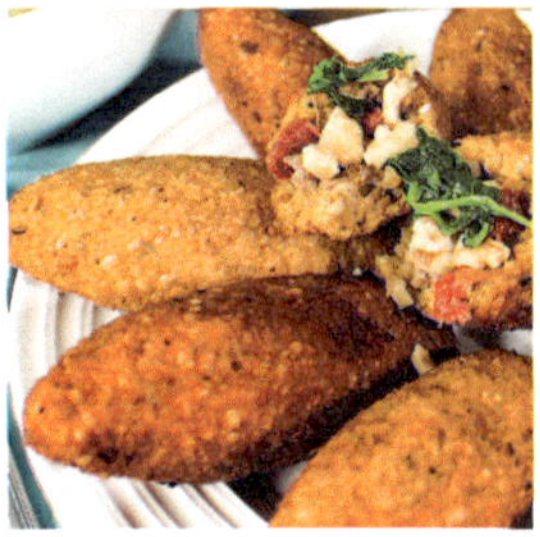

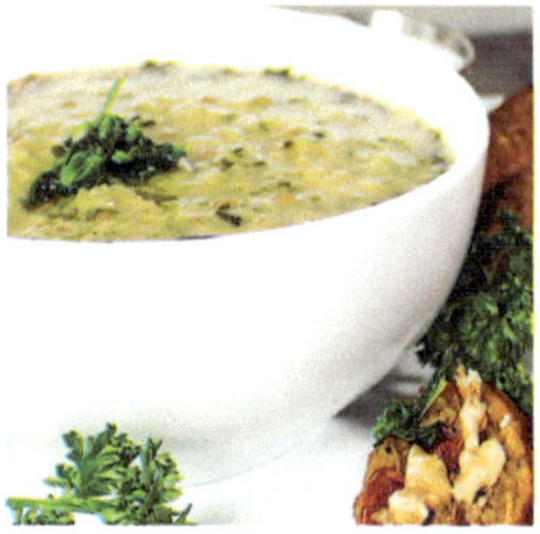

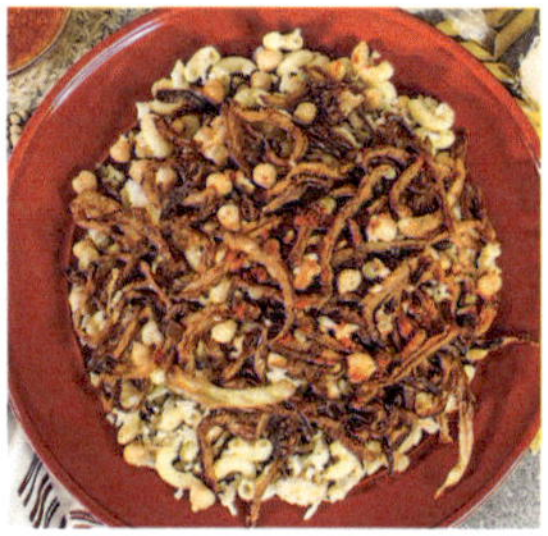

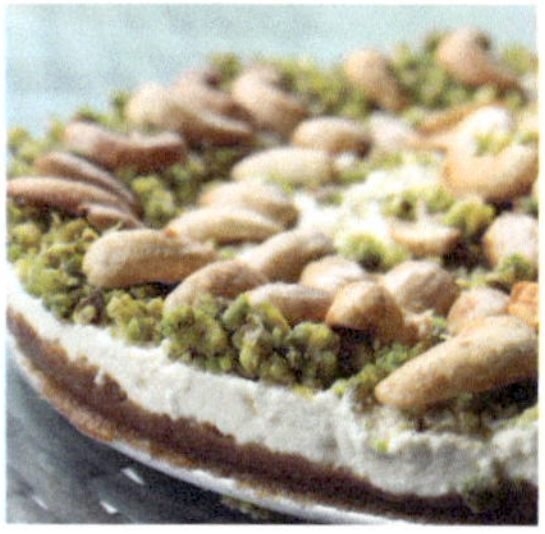

AN A-Z OF RESOURCES FOR VEGANS

This section is from the notes I've kept over the years as I've researched non-animal-based resources for vegans. Most of these entries detail the effects various plants, seeds, nuts, and fungi have, where they came from, and how they may taste. People I've met over the years thought it would be useful for me to include these notes in this book, so here they are!

It's not really an "A-Z" (my editor, graphic designer, and I kept referring to it like that, and I liked it, so that's what we called it here) because it's not an exhaustive list—these are notes I've taken and refined and that I now hope can help you as you start exploring veganism. Hopefully, you read about something and do some research about how you can involve it in your journey. Going vegan is partially an exploration of food and health, and the more you learn about it, the more informed you tend to get about your diet. It's good to learn about what you put into your body!

Please remember, I'm not a doctor, and I'm certainly not your doctor. Do not use any of the home remedies listed in the following pages if you have any medical conditions that could be triggered or worsened by those ingredients.

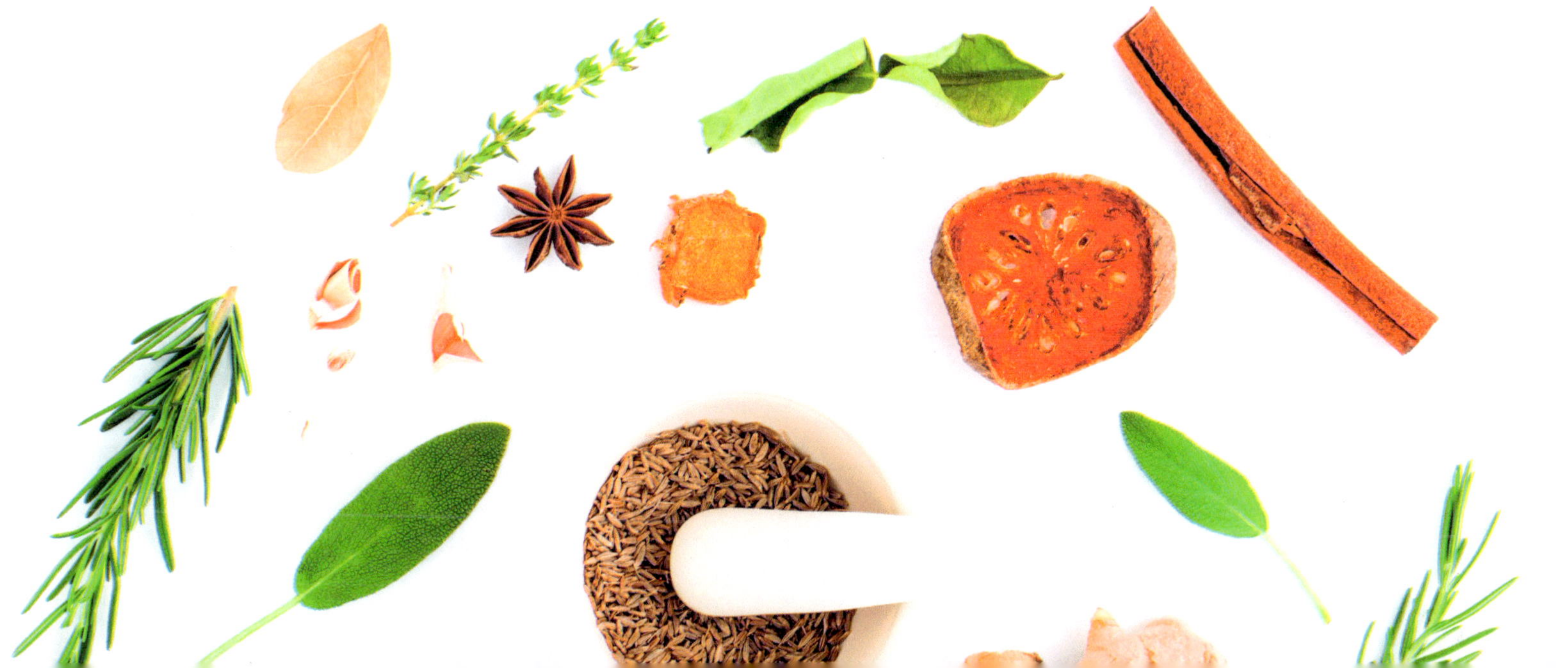

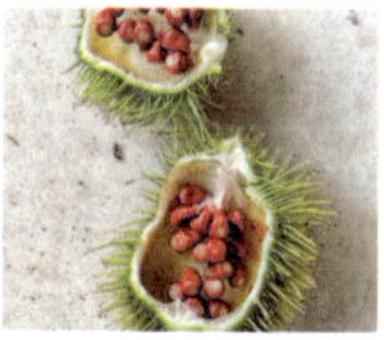

ACHIOTE

Source of annatto, a natural orange-red substance used in Latin American and Caribbean dishes and as an industrial food coloring to add color to many products. It has amino acids, iron, phosphorus, beta-carotene, vitamin C, and hypoglycemic properties. Its roots reduce blood glucose levels, and tea steeped from the leaves helps alleviate digestive problems, including diarrhea and the symptoms of dysentery.

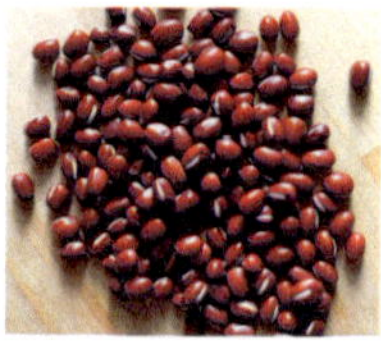

ADZUKI

Sometimes referred to as the red mung bean, it comes from Asia. Usually red, but white, black, gray, and variously mottled varieties. High in fiber and protein. It helps treat bladder infections and urinary dysfunction in both men and women. Adzuki can play a role in losing weight due to the bulkiness it provides our stomachs to feel full for longer. Due to the high protein, it can help to keep sugar levels low.

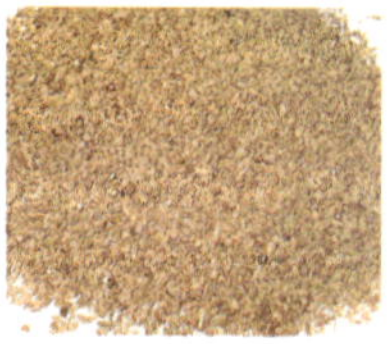

AJWAIN

The small, oval-shaped, pale brown seed-like fruits, like caraway, cumin, and fennel, have a flavor similar to anise and oregano and smell close to thyme. Rich in fiber, minerals, vitamins, and antioxidants, it can help the digestive function of the intestinal tract, easing flatulence and indigestion. The oil can act as local an anesthetic, anti-bacterial, and antifungal.

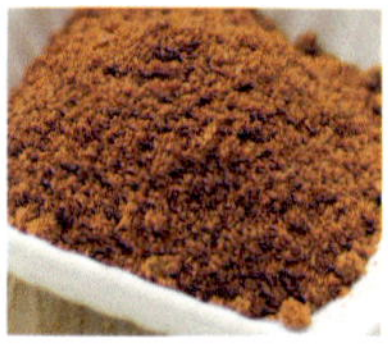

ALLSPICE

A spice the English thought combined the flavors of cinnamon, nutmeg, and clove. It can improve digestion and ease issues such as diarrhea and nausea. Its oil may help kill disease-causing germs on food. It seems to help resist against infectious agents, has local anesthetic and antiseptic properties, and increases blood flow (making the skin feel warmer).

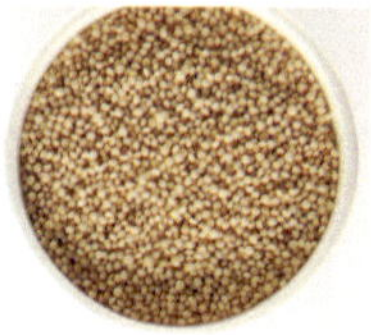

AMARANTH

A blanket word for many plants in the amaranthus genus, when we talk about "amaranth," we mean the grain. It's packed with vitamins and minerals and is referred to as "the ultimate meat substitute." It contains no gluten but can contain phytochemicals that may act as antinutrients, but cooking decreases their effects.

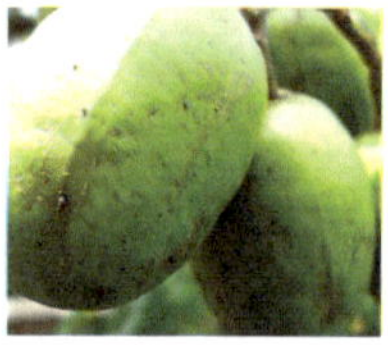

AMBARELLA

Also known as a "June plum" and dozens of other names across multiple tropical regions. This is an almost magical fruit because people use it to treat diabetes, indigestion, urinary tract infections, hypertension, inflamed hemorrhoids, sores, wounds, and burns. The leaves and bark treat other diseases, including dysentery and thrush.

A

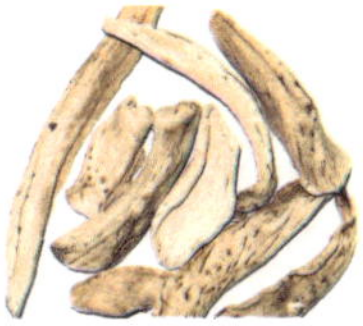

AMCHOOR

A spice powder made from dried green mangoes, it brings much of the fruit's benefits with it. It has been a mainstay in Indian cuisine for over 4,000 years. It is said to control blood pressure and diabetes, maintain heart health, and possibly have anti-cancer properties. If you have an allergy to mangoes, consuming amchoor can result in a reaction and even anaphylaxis.

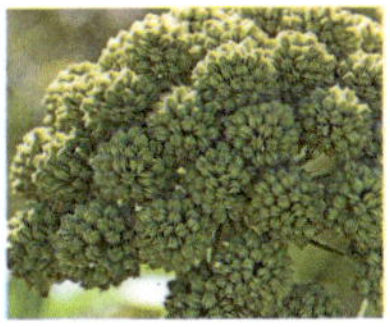

ANGELICA

Growing wild across northern Europe, the roots, stems, and seeds have been used for food and medicine for centuries. It's been used to treat heartburn, gas, nausea, vomiting, diarrhea, and many other things. Avoid if you have diabetes, are pregnant, are breastfeeding, are oftne exposed to the sun or taking blood thinners.

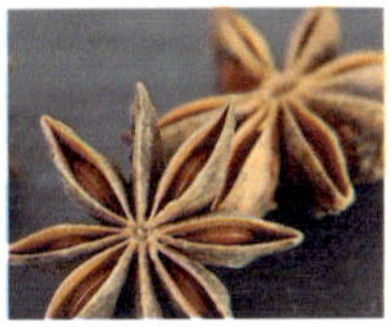

ANISE

Many think this is licorice, and the taste is similar, but it's a different plant. Contains calcium, iron, copper, potassium, manganese, zinc, and magnesium and can help control blood pressure, boost blood production, stimulate blood circulation, and promotes digestion. Its seeds may also increase libido and bring relief from coughing.

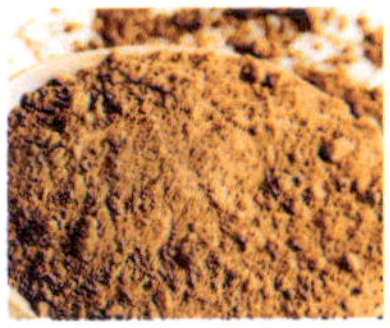

ANNATTO

(See Achiote)

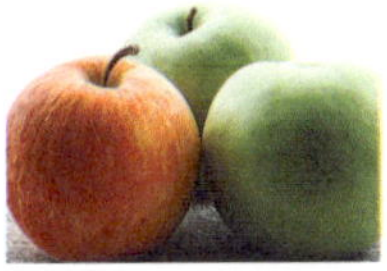

APPLE

"An apple a day keeps the doctor away" isn't all wrong. Most varieties (both eating and cooking) of apples can supply an amazing amount of vitamins C and B6, and it's high in potassium. Its high fiber content is excellent for your GI tract, and it's rich in antioxidants that protect the body and cells from damaging free radicals.

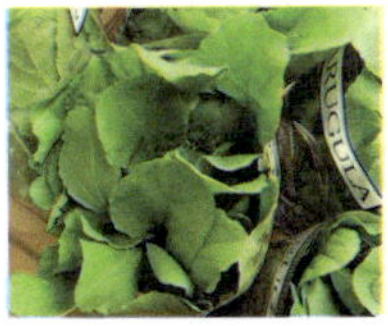

ARUGULA

A leafy, lettuce-like vegetable grown across the Mediterranean and regularly used in salads or on sandwiches or pizza. It is rich in antioxidants, which can help protect against cancer. Also an excellent source of folate and other B vitamins, vitamins C and K, and potassium. If you are on blood thinners, avoid overeatin.

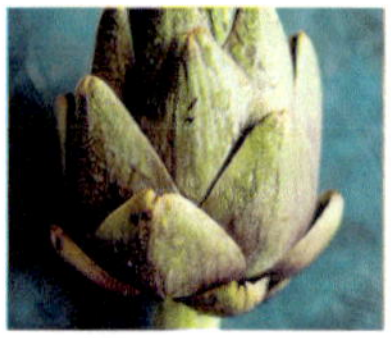

ARTICHOKE

A Mediterranean thistle, but we usually don't see it in full bloom. It's been food, medicine, and tea for many centuries. It can aid in digestion (possibly aiding irritable bowel syndrome), there is research showing it may lower cholesterol, and the flower head has one of the largest antioxidant capacities in all vegetables.

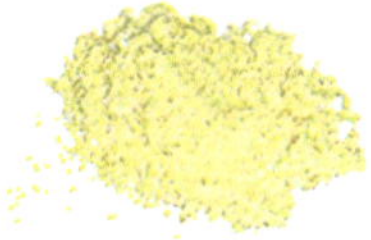

ASAFOETIDA

A latex that comes from the roots of several ferulas (part of the celery family) across Iran, Afghanistan, and parts of the Indian subcontinent. It has a strong smell which dissipates after cooking. It's heavily used as a flavor enhancer in dishes like curries, and regularly used to relive gas and menstrual cramps.

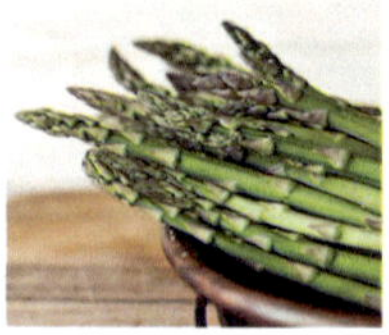

ASPARAGUS

It was once a delicacy—the Romans had a fleet to haul it—and fresh asparagus is still popular in Europe. It's a great source of vitamins B1, B2, B9 (folate), and iron, and loaded with vitamin K. And that smell? It's sulfur-containing compounds breaking down as you digest it (not everyone can smell it, though!).

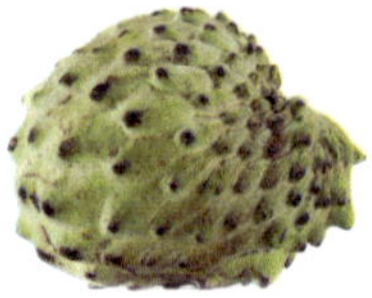

ATEMOYA

A hybrid of the sugar-apple and the cherimoya, this is juicy, (sometimes overly) sweet tropical fruit. It is rich in protein, carbohydrates, vitamin A, phosphorous, and calcium. It may help with weight control, lower cholesterol, lower blood pressure, and it may help reduce the risk of cancers and heart disease. The seeds are toxic and should be removed when eating.

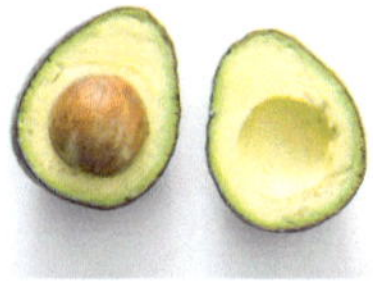

AVOCADO

A fruit (a very large berry) from a Latin American tree of the same name. Usually served sliced or in guacamole, the leaves are sometimes used as a spice. The fruit provides a lot of B5, B6, and folate, in addition it also delivers a lot of vitamin K, potassium, fat, and even some protein. The leaves, bark, skin, pit, and even fruit are harmful to many animals.

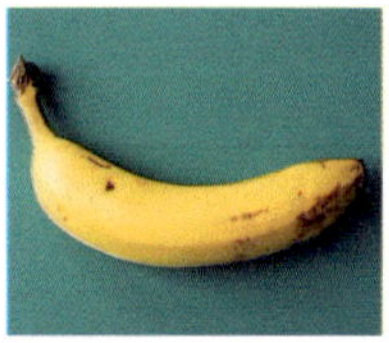

BANANA

A botanical berry. The starchier varieties are referred to as "plantains" and are cooked in savory dishes (tostones are amazing!). When eaten in moderation, bananas are likely to help cholesterol levels and are helpful in lowering blood pressure. They're an excellent source of potassium and dietary fiber, but keep an eye on their glycemic index.

B

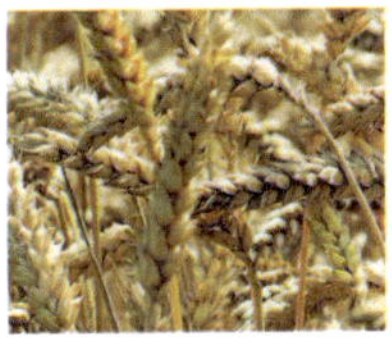

BARLEY

A grass and major cereal grain, barley has been cultivated by humans for 10,000 years. Barley can support large populations of good bacteria, is high in niacin and other B vitamins (not heavy on the folate, though). At least six servings of whole grains a week eating is a great idea, especially for postmenopausal women with high cholesterol, high blood pressure, or other signs of cardiovascular disease.

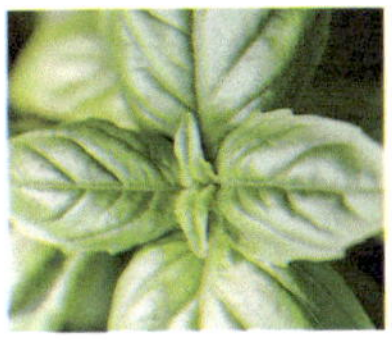

BASIL

An annual and native to central Africa and Southeast Asia, basil has many therapeutic properties in folk medicines. The seeds are used in various drinks, and the essential oil shows antifungal (though it can be susceptible to crop-devastating fungi) and insect-repelling properties (including being toxic to mosquitos). Very high in many vitamins, iron, and manganese.

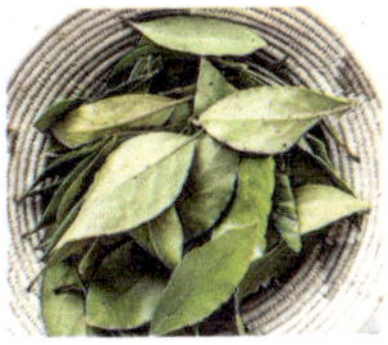

BAY LEAF

Widespread in many cuisines, it's rich in vitamins and minerals—except you should only eat it if it's been ground, as the leaf, when dry, is extremely sharp and can cause choking or even bleeding along your GI tract. It has various medicinal uses (as an astringent and diuretic), can be an appetite stimulant, and also has insect repellent properties.

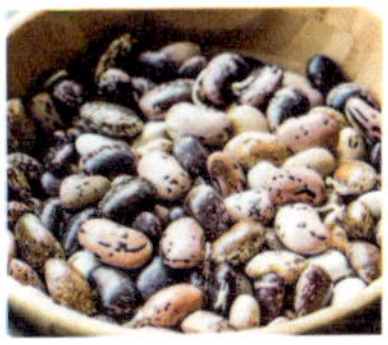

BEAN

Providing protein, complex carbohydrates, vitamins, fiber, and iron, beans are a cornerstone of a vegan diet. Anasazi, black beans, black-eyed peas, chickpeas, and soy beans (see Soy for more information) are often found in yummy recipes. Just cook them fully, as otherwise they can be toxic or infected with bacteria. Some can inhibit bone growth and interfere with vitamin D metabolism.

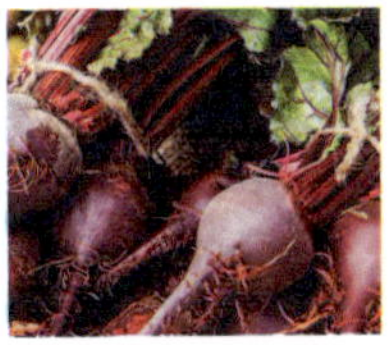

BEET

What Americans think of as a "beet" is beetroot—the taproot of a beet plant. The entire beet is edible and nutritious (the greens being as nutritious as kale), and the roots have been found to provide antioxidant and anti-inflammatory properties, as well as being an excellent source of folate. Those with kidney or gallbladder problems may want to avoid eating beet greens.

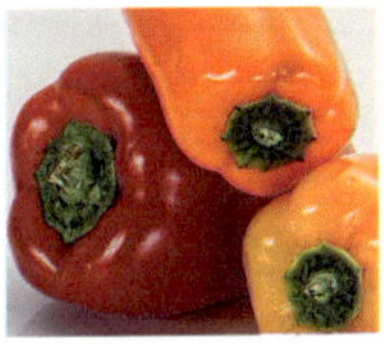

BELL PEPPER

The common everyday pepper is the only member of its family that doesn't produce capsaicin (the chemical that makes peppers burn). It is very high in vitamin C (the red ones having twice the amount than the green), and high in A (the red ones, not the green) and B6 (not much else, though). They are thought to aid digestion, may help eyesight, and have anti-inflammatory properties. Avoid it if they cause you tummy trouble.

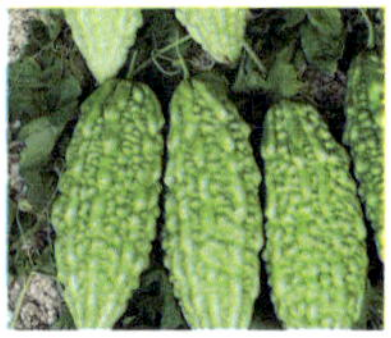

BITTER MELON

Named for its bitter taste, this subtropical fruit is found in the regional cuisines of southeast Asia, China, India, and other surrounding areas. It has been used in many folk medicines over the years, but the primary benefit seems to be lowering blood glucose levels in diabetics. It can cause temporary side effects, such as abdominal trouble, and should not be consumed by pregnant women.

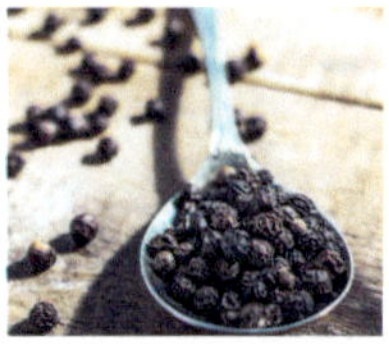

BLACK PEPPER

4,000 years ago in India, the peppercorn was a prized trade good. It was believed to cure abscesses, toothaches, sunburn—even insomnia! It has decent amounts of vitamin K, iron, and manganese, and is thought to be most beneficial by increasing absorption of selenium, beta-carotene, and vitamin B12. Large amounts are unsafe for children or when pregnant, and it can adversely affect those with diabetes and bleeding disorders.

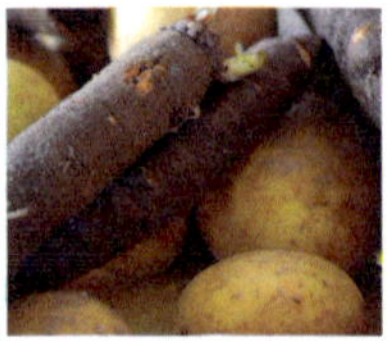

BLACK SALSIFY

Also known as the "vegetable oyster" because it tastes like a saltwater mollusk. Fairly nutritious, it contains protein (about 6% of your recommended daily allowance) and is high in carbohydrates, riboflavin, vitamin C, manganese, phosphorus, potassium, sodium. It's also a bit sweet and used in a crystalized dessert in Portugal.

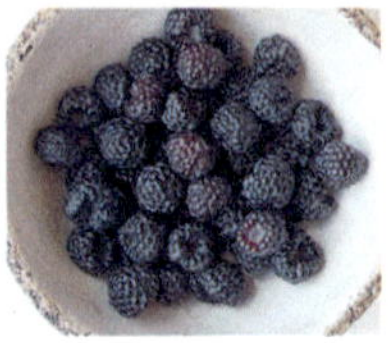

BLACKBERRY

A sweet berry common in Europe and North America, used for snacking, in desserts, or in jellies and jams. They're extremely high in vitamins C and K, with good levels of folate, vitamin E, iron, magnesium, and zinc. The leaves have been used medicinally since ancient times, usually by chewing or using the shoots for a tea used to treat sore throats, thrush, and diarrhea.

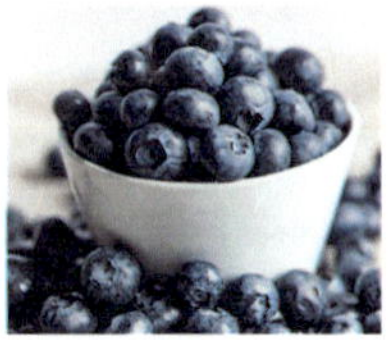

BLUEBERRY

A common berry in North America, used mostly for snacking, jams, and jellies. Low in calories, it's rich in vitamins C and K and manganese. It's currently under research as it is high in antioxidants that can protect you against free radicals. It seems to lower blood pressure and reduce cholesterol, may have an anti-diabetes effect, and may even counter the DNA damage that leads to aging.

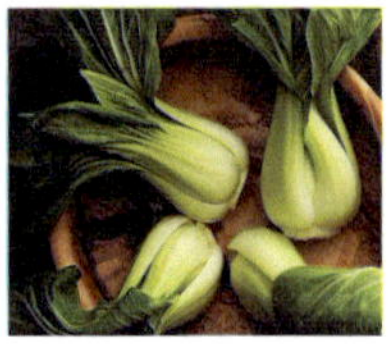

BOK CHOY

A cabbage popular in southern China and Southeast Asia, but also hardy in the winter, so it's growing in popularity in the northern hemisphere. Massively rich in vitamins A, B6, C, K, beta-Carotene, and calcium. While one of the most nutrient-rich foods available, it also contains glucosinolates, which are possibly able to help prevent cancer in small doses, can be toxic in very large doses.

B

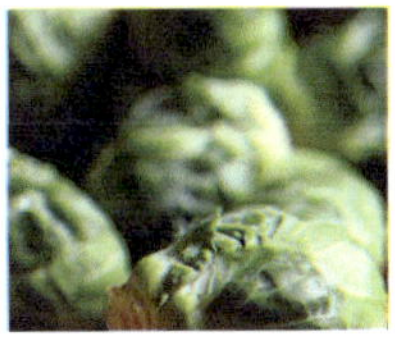

BRUSSELS SPROUT

A budding cabbage popular in Belgium (which may be the reason for its name). It contains over 100% of the recommended vitamins C and K, and is high in many of the B vitamins along with iron, manganese, and phosphorous. Despite their benefits, eating them in excess is not recommended for those on blood thinners, as vitamin K is a blood-clotting factor.

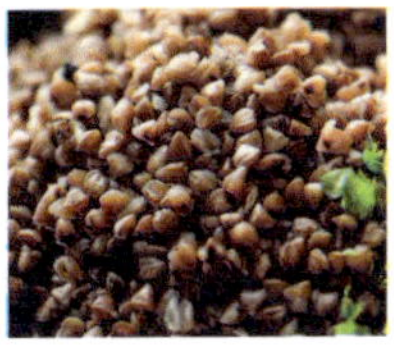

BUCKWHEAT

It's possible we have been cultivating buckwheat for 8,000 years (starting in Asia). Nutritionally, it is especially high in riboflavin, niacin, pantothenic acid, vitamin B6, iron, magnesium, manganese, phosphorous, and zinc. It may help against hardening of the arteries, increase blood flow and circulation issues. Those with gluten sensitivities or allergies to rice or latex should avoid it.

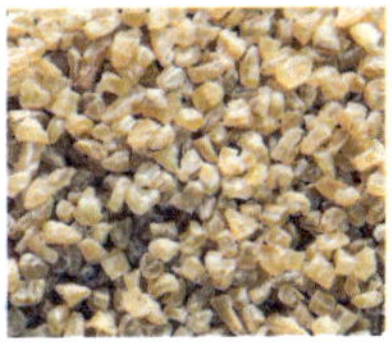

BULGUR

Often confused with cracked wheat, bulgur is cracked parboiled wheat groats. It's used a lot in this book, and for good reason. It's not a nutrient powerhouse (though it is high in manganese), but it's high in fiber. The fiber is the reason it may be good for your heart, blood sugar, digestive health, and might help with weight loss (like most whole grains). Avoid it if you have issues with gluten or other GI disorders.

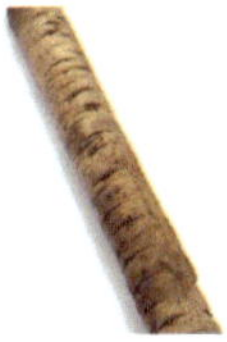

BURDOCK

Related to the artichoke, the stalks and leaves can be consumed when the plant is young, and the taproot is used in many ways. Contains a decent amount of calcium, potassium, amino acids. Pregnant women should avoid it, but it may encourage lactation in breastfeeding women. The plant contains lactones which can cause contact dermatitis in those who are allergic. Turks also say it wards off the "evil eye."

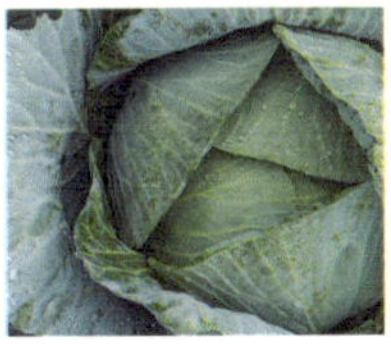

CABBAGE

There is no clinical evidence cabbage (including its cousin red cabbage) has medicinal effects, however, its effects on diseases (including colon cancer) are being studied. It is very rich in vitamins C and K, and strong in B6, folate, and dietary fiber. Traditionally, the juice and mashed cabbage have been used to treat many things, such as mushroom poisoning and ulcers, but it can also cause painful gas in some.

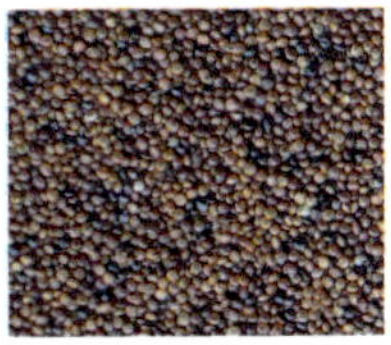

CAÑIHUA

Also known as "kaniwa," this is a Andean goosefoot is closely related to quinoa, but less bitter. It is high in protein and dietary fiber. Like many of the indigenous food crops of that region, not only is its protein content higher than most cereals, the calcium, zinc, and iron is, too. It can be milled into flour. There are little-to-no known side effects, as this is not a wheat and those with gluten intolerances should be able to eat it safely.

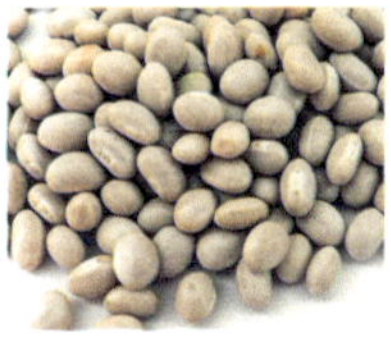

CANNELLINI

Also known as the white kidney bean, it is thought to have originated in South America, then spreading to become a staple in the Mediterranean and parts of Asia. They can help reduce blood sugar, fight diabetes due to their high fiber, and may help fight cancer due to their high antioxidants. While not as toxic as red kidney beans, they should still always be fully cooked before consuming.

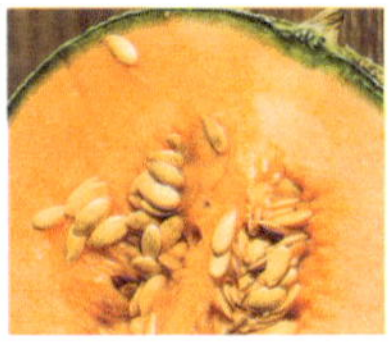

CANTALOUPE

This sweet, orange-fleshed muskmelon is versatile, used for snacks, desserts, or a counterpart to savory flavors in dishes. A raw melon is 90% water, with its primary nutrient being vitamin C, followed by large amounts of vitamin A and beta-Carotene. The surface can hold harmful bacteria from the soil (including salmonella), so ensure it's thoroughly washed before cutting.

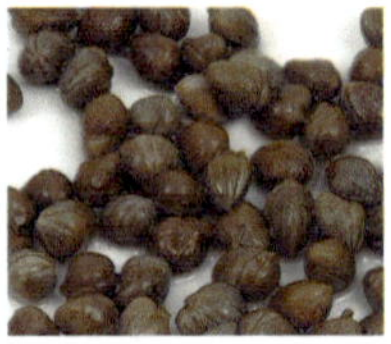

CAPER

The bud of the caper bush, we usually eat these pickled and preserved. Packed with iron, vitamins K and B2 (riboflavin), it also has antioxidant properties. In ancient times, it was used to alleviate gas, and in Biblical times, the berry was said to be an aphrodisiac. A serving of preserved capers can contain close to 200% of your daily allowance of sodium, so use sparingly.

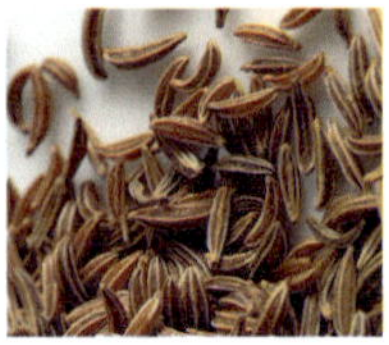

CARAWAY

We eat what we think are seeds but are actually the fruit. The use of caraway goes back to ancient times, treating flatulence and indigestion in traditional medicines, though it is now mostly recognized for its essential oils. It is very high in minerals (though low in sodium) and vitamins. It seems to have some side effects for pregnant women and diabetics.

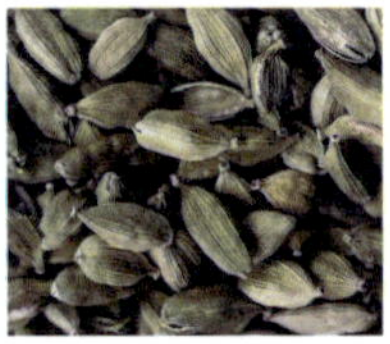

CARDAMOM

A spice used heavily in food and beverages across the world. It is one of the three most expensive spices (vanilla and saffron being the other two) and used for its essential oils (which require care in storage). Studies have shown anti-microbial and anti-cancer effects, as well helping fight metabolic syndromes. Medicinal amounts may not be healthy for pregnant women.

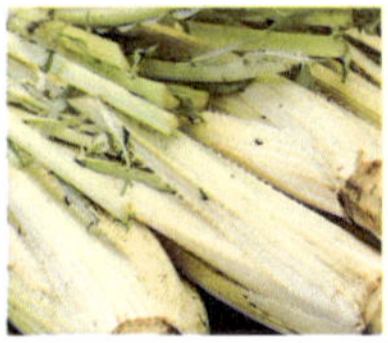

CARDOON

A thistle in the sunflower family, the earliest mention of this artichoke-like plant goes is from ancient times. Its late seasonality means it is sometimes a staple for dinners during northern hemisphere winter holidays. It has moderate levels of folate, magnesium, manganese, and potassium, but is high in sodium. It seems to have mild laxative properties and cholesterol-lowering effects.

C

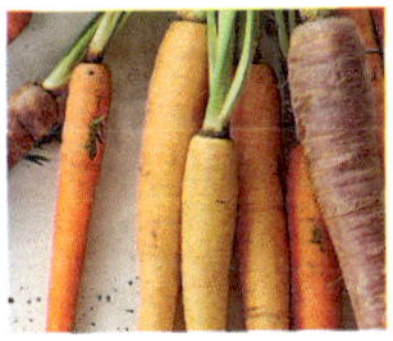

CARROTS

This root won't better your vision (unless you have a vitamin A deficiency). They're high in vitamin A equivalents, strong in vitamins B6 and K, contain some dietary fiber, and may have anti-cancer properties. Young children should avoid the juice (it can decay their teeth and affect their skin color), and those with "celery-carrot-mugwort-spice syndrome" may have an allergic reaction.

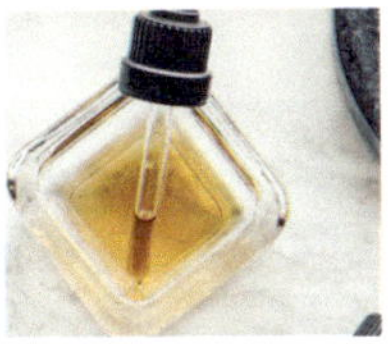

CASSIA

The ground bark of an evergreen native to south Asia, this is what we usually consume as cinnamon (see cinnamon for more). Its essential oil is what gives it its taste and its health benefits (the Chinese consider it a fundamental herb in traditional medicine), and it may have anti-cancer effects and help fight prediabetes and other conditions. It can be toxic to humans in high amounts.

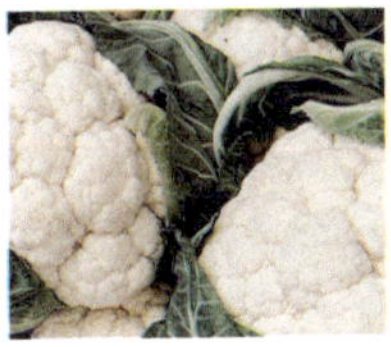

CAULIFLOWER

A member of the mustard family, this plant is related to other "cole" crops, such as Brussels sprouts, cabbage, and kale. The first mentions of it go back almost 2,000 years. It has very high levels of vitamin C and moderate ones of several B vitamins and vitamin K. It is also rich in good phytochemicals and is being researched for their benefits.

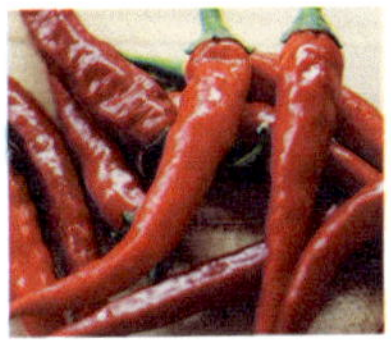

CAYENNE PEPPER

A moderately hot chili pepper, it is used to introduce spice to a dish (either whole or in its powdered form). It is rich in antioxidants and the capsaicin found within it can ease psoriasis, aid in digestive health, and possibly reduce cancer and blood pressure risks. Like any hot pepper, it can cause discomfort if too many are consumed. It may also interact with blood thinners and other medications.

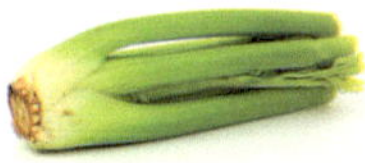

CELERY

A plant that has been harvested going back into antiquity. Its seed can be used as a spice, and its extracts are used in herbal medicine (celery salt, for example, is used to treat joint pain and gout). Rich in vitamin K, it is over 95% water, but provides low-calorie dietary fiber, and is used in many weight loss diets. Celery can cause fatal anaphylactic shock, so be aware of any allergic reactions.

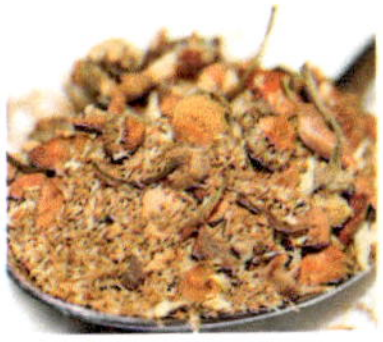

CHAMOMILE

This daisy-like plant is said to address GI issues, anxiety, insomnia, and migraines—and even using tea bags as compresses to relieve eye strain. However, its polyphenol compounds can cause miscarriage and interactions with anticoagulants, aspirin, and other drugs. Those with ragweed allergies, or who have had endometriosis, uterine fibroids, or cancers of the breast, ovary, and uterus should avoid it.

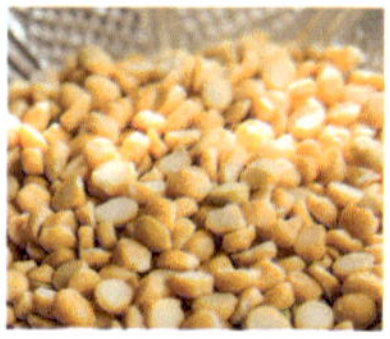

CHANA DAL

A popular preparation for black chickpeas in India, this is high in protein, folate, manganese, and dietary fiber. It is often used in soups, but many other preparations, including snacks like dholka and vada, are also common. A dal dish fills you for several hours and can help to reduce snacking between meals.

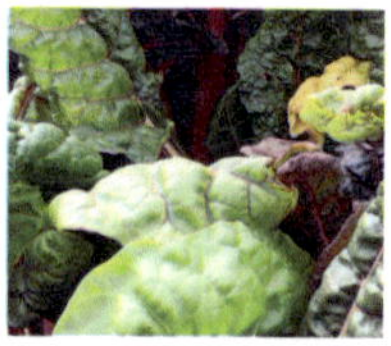

CHARD

Sometimes called "swiss chard," it isn't Swiss. Used in salads, soups, and more, it's a good source of nutrients—vitamin E, magnesium, manganese, iron, and potassium, along moderate levels of other nutrients. It's high in antioxidants, works as an anti-cancer agent, regulates sugar, and helps maintain healthy eyes and nervous system. There are oxalates here, so those with kidney or gallstones should avoid it.

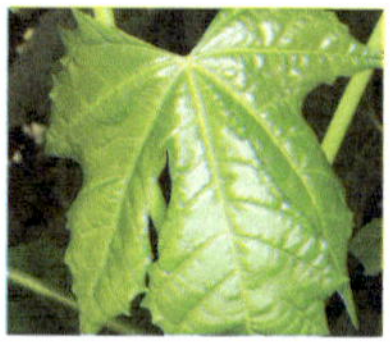

CHAYA

Also known as "tree spinach," these leaves have quite a few health benefits when cooked (vitamins A and B1, ascorbic acid, iron, calcium, phosphorus, protein, carbohydrates, and antioxidants are all to be found). Uncooked leaves produce hydrogen cyanide when they're damaged, handling the plant long-term can result in irritation or an allergic reaction, and cooking in aluminum can result in a toxic reaction.

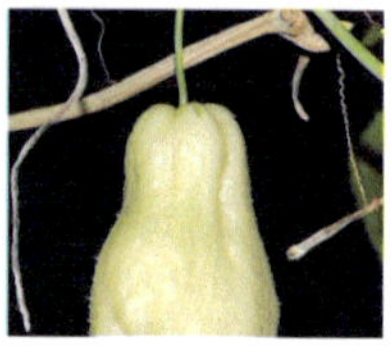

CHAYOTE

A roughly pear-shaped gourd originating from South America, this plant is fully edible (though most only know it for the fruit). Most find the raw fruit to be unpalatable, so it is usually cooked. An excellent source of folate, it is also high in vitamin C and zinc. Some people experience irritation when their skin is exposed to the peeled fruit.

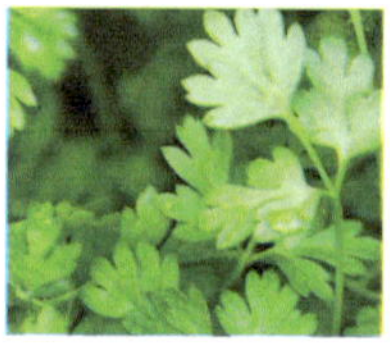

CHERVIL

Popular in various folk medicine, this herb is mostly used as a flavoring agent. Some find it helpful with gout, skin conditions, high blood pressure, and digestion issues. There are no known drug interactions, but in high doses it may interfere in development of the fetus during pregnancy.

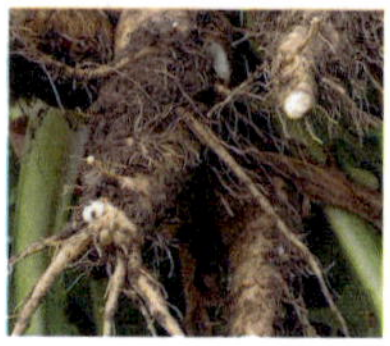

CHICORY

Your relatives who lived during World War II might not like this—it was used to cut the coffee supply and make it stretch (but those who enjoy a New Orleans-style vegetarian café au lait likely love it). It may help with gall bladder issues, high blood pressure, and constipation. However, it may lower blood sugar and stimulate bile production. Those allergic to ragweed should avoid it.

C

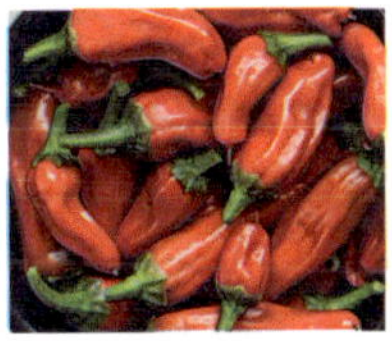

CHILI PEPPER

A term for 50,000 varieties of fruits in the genus Capsicum. Their varying spiciness, vitamin B6, and the vitamin C and beta-carotene many provide make them vital in food and medicine. They can relieve nerve pain, nausea, cluster headaches, and other issues. Those with diabetes, high blood pressure, or a bleeding disorder should stay away from a lot of capsicum.

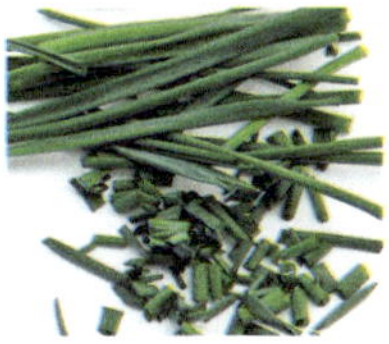

CHIVES

With cultivation dating back 5,000 years, this is a perennial that produces edible leaves, flowers, and stalks used heavily as ingredients in many dishes. Romans believed it could act as a diuretic, but now, we recognize it for its abundant vitamins C and k, folate, iron, magnesium, and manganese. There are little to no side effects, but too much can upset a stomach.

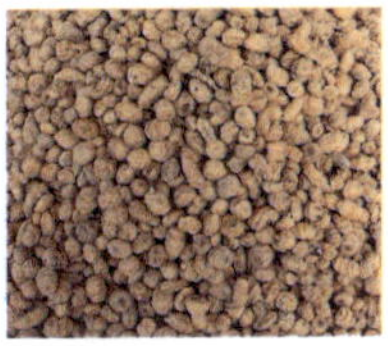

CHUFA

A sedge with an edible tuber that is also referred to as the "tiger nut." Rich in vitamins C and E, is also a good source of reliable calcium, phosphorus, magnesium, potassium, and iron. While it's been cultivated for thousands of years, most would know it in the drink horchata at this point. It has been used to relieve diarrhea and indigestion traditionally.

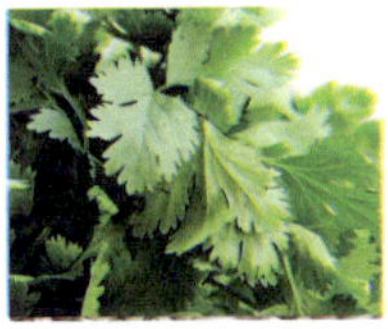

CILANTRO

(See Coriander)

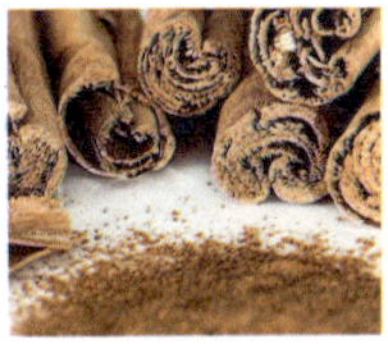

CINNAMON

Real cinnamon (see Cassia for what we typically consume as cinnamon) has been a prized spice and aromatic going back into antiquity and used the world over in numerous ways. It's rich in many vitamins and minerals, and has long been used as a digestive aid. Too much can result in gastrointestinal disorders and allergic reactions.

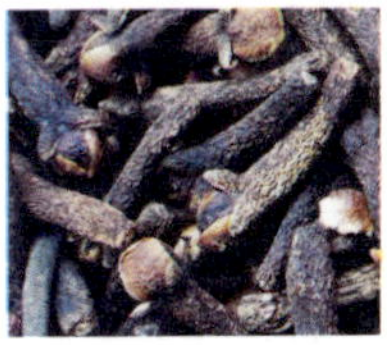

CLOVES

The flower buds of trees native to Indonesia, this has long been used in Asian and Latin American cuisines and traditional medicine. In traditional uses, it has been used for toothaches, fever reduction, premature ejaculation, and even as an insect repellent. The FDA warns those with liver disease, blood clotting and immune system disorders, and food allergies to stay away from it.

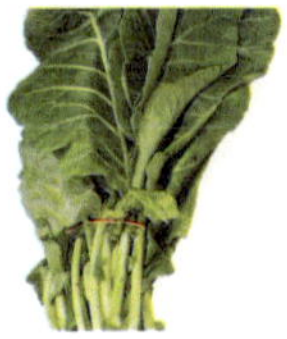

COLLARD

Loose-leafed cultivars (with large, dark green leaves) of the same family cabbage and broccoli come from. It's been consumed for over 2,000 years across multiple continents and is a staple in the southern cuisine of the US. Massively high in vitamin K, it's also rich in vitamin A equivalents, beta-Carotene, vitamin C, calcium, and manganese.

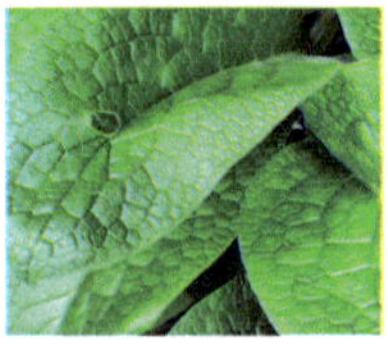

COMFREY

A genus of flowering plants used in gardening and traditional medicine. In herbal medicine it is used topically and has traditionally been used to help mend bone after a break. High in minerals and vitamins, it is supposedly good in expelling mucus and lowering cholesterol but is highly toxic to the liver (the FDA banned it in 2001 for internal use in the US).

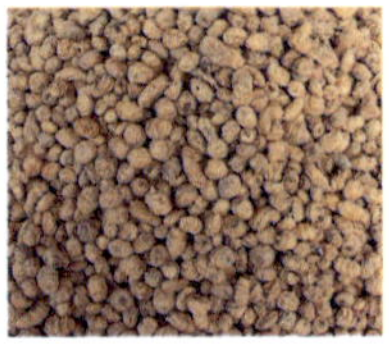

CORIANDER

An annual herb that is fully edible, though we tend to eat the fresh leaves (cilantro) or the seeds (which are referred to as coriander). It is cultivated over Asia and southern Europe, with evidence of it being used going back at least 2,00 years. The leaves are heavily rich in vitamin K, and a great source of numerous other vitamins and minerals.

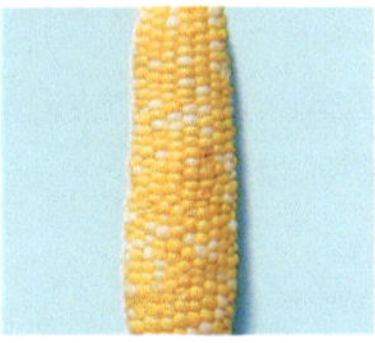

CORN

A cereal otherwise known as "maize," corn comes from people 10,000 years ago in what is now Mexico. Over the centuries, it has spread across the word, and many varieties have been developed. Corn's uses are wide and varied, but as a food, it's rich in vitamins B1, B3, B5, B9 (folate), and magnesium and phosphorus, while also delivering some protein and dietary fiber.

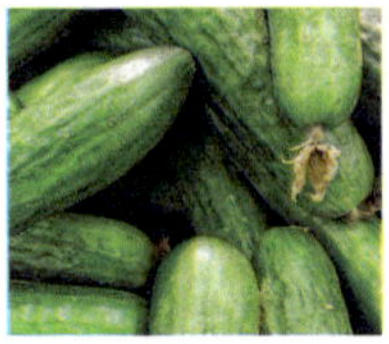

CUCUMBER

The fruit of a creeping vine that is commonly used as a vegetable. Originating in India, and being brought back to Europe by the Greeks or the Romans, it has been cultivated around the world. It's not heavily rich in nutrition, though it does have quite a bit of vitamin K. It is used in numerous ways, including pickling. It has been used for urinary issues, high and low blood pressure, and may be beneficial to those with diabetes.

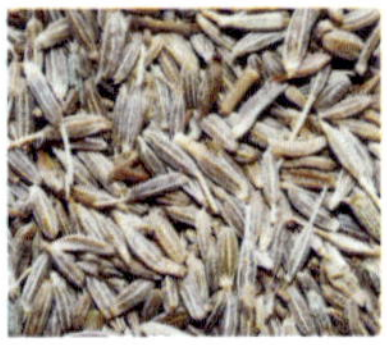

CUMIN

The seeds from the herb's fruit are dried and ground, giving us the spice with the same name. Very rich in most of the B vitamins (though not in folate) and vitamin K, it's also an excellent source of many minerals (including calcium, iron, magnesium, manganese, phosphorus, and potassium). Research shows it may reduce cholesterol and improve weight loss in some. It may slow clotting and lower blood sugar too far, so avoid it in those cases.

E

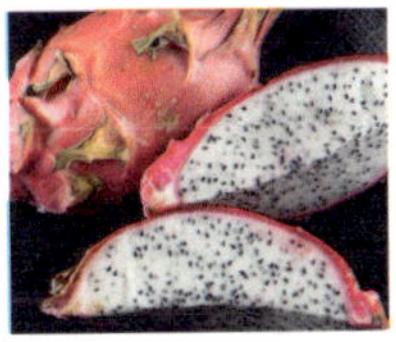

DRAGON FRUIT

These are the fruit of several tropical and sub-tropical cacti. The seeds are strong in oils, and especially strong in palmitic, oleic, and linoleic acids and are a good source of vitamin C and calcium. The fruit's texture is like a kiwi, and the flowers can be eaten or steeped in tea. There is little research done on them, but it seems standard levels of consumption have no ill effects, and higher doses seem to lower blood sugar levels in those with prediabetes.

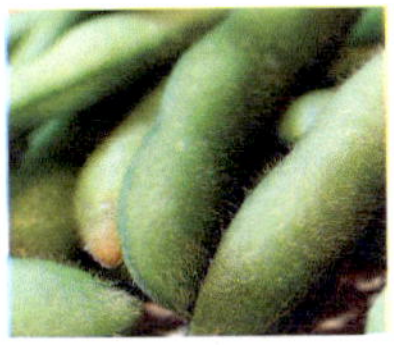

EDAMAME

(See Soy)

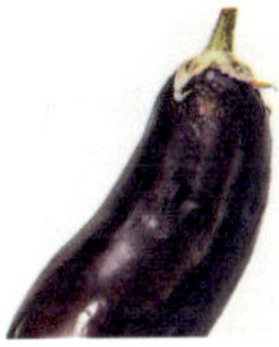

EGGPLANT

Either originating in India or Africa, the eggplant is technically a berry. Traditionally, it was said to cause insanity and considered poisonous (which the leaves, when eaten in large quantities, are). It's common in various world cuisines, making it easy to find recipes for it. It provides numerous vitamins and minerals, and because of that, it is ideal for numerous health conditions (including diabetes and possibly cancer).

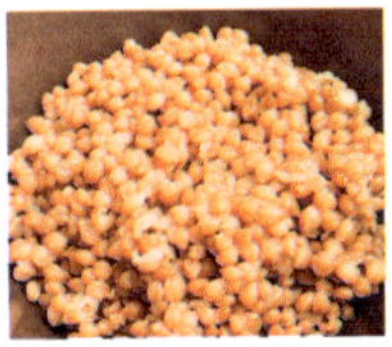

EINKORN

A wheat, but not just any wheat. It originated from the Fertile Crescent and is one of the first domesticated plants in human history. It's low-yielding, but tolerant of poor or dry soil. It's more nutritious than most modern wheats as it has higher levels of fat, protein, and various vitamins and minerals and is where bulgur typically comes from. It does still include gluten, so those with an intolerance should avoid it.

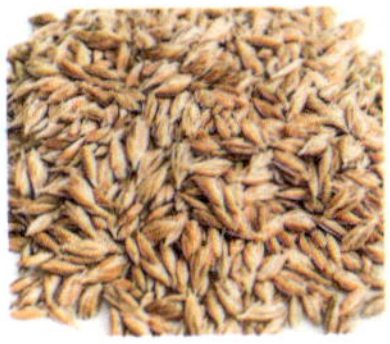

EMMER

Another early domesticated wheat from the Fertile Crescent, this is mostly consumed by humans (while einkorn is also used in animal feed) and is considered to make good bread. Emmer is mostly found wild and in mountainous regions now, but is becoming very popular in various European markets, being used in "luxury" breads and baked goods, and is grown in India as it is hardy and drought resistant.

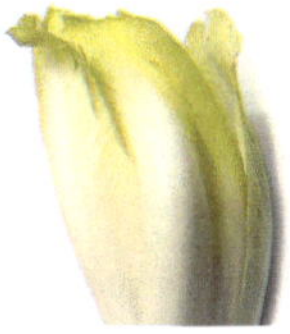

ENDIVE

Part of chicory's family, there are two main types—curly endive (often confused for chicory in the USA) and escarole. Very rich in vitamin K and manganese, it's also a good source for folate, B5, vitamin A equivalent, and beta-Carotene. It's usually cooked like other greens or in stews. Those on blood thinners should avoid it due to its large amount of vitamin K, and there are some reports of allergies.

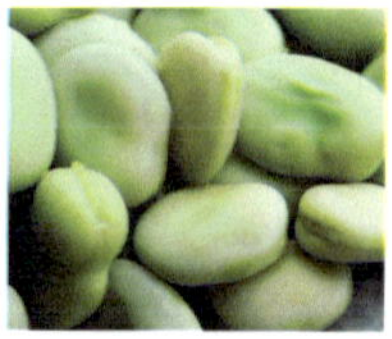

FAVA

Also referred to as "broad beans," fava are wide ranging and come from a relatively unknown origin. While one of Hannibal Lecter's favorite sides, they have also been used as a laxative, a non-animal-based manure, and are heavily nutritious in almost all of the major vitamins and minerals. However, these need to be prepared correctly as they are toxic (boiling them for 10 minutes will destroy the toxic substance).

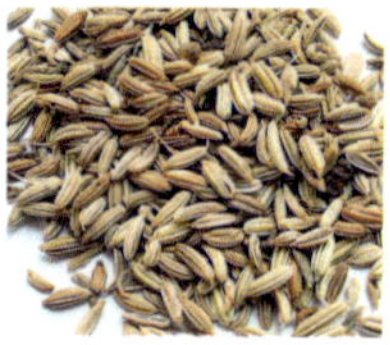

FENNEL

A hardy, flowering, aromatic plant that is part of the carrot family. It originates from the Mediterranean-but has adapted well across the world. It is used heavily in alcoholic drinks (notably absinthe), is remarkably rich in most vitamins and minerals, and may ease colic in babies and menstrual or menopausal symptoms. It is possibly unsafe when breastfeeding, and those with allergies to celery, carrot, or mugwort should avoid it.

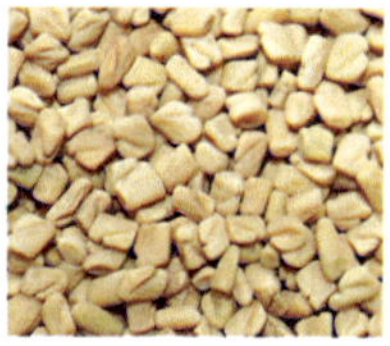

FENUGREEK

While rich in protein and many vitamins and minerals, take caution with fenugreek. It was once a folk remedy for increasing mother's milk production, though research is inconclusive on its ability to do so, is used in Indian and Turkish cuisines, and in Ethiopia, it has been said to ease diabetes (though it also seems to cause hypoglycemia in those individuals).

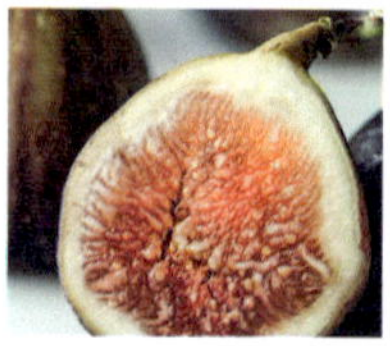

FIG

The "fruit" of a fiscus tree, the common fig isn't really a fruit at all—it's many small flowers growing within an inverted, closed receptacle. A good source of many vitamins and minerals, initial research show their phytochemicals may have benefits in dealing with high cholesterol, and traditionally the tree's sap has been used to soften calluses and remove warts.

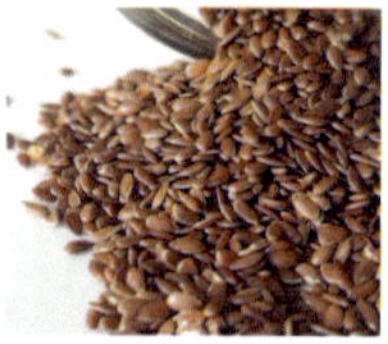

FLAXSEED

Used in various applications, flaxseed has strong health benefits delivered alongside its high nutritional content (especially the B vitamins, iron, magnesium, and phosphorus), including helping with cholesterol, dealing with body weight, and reducing high blood pressure. Freshly ground flaxseed can go rancid within a week, so be aware of that if using it.

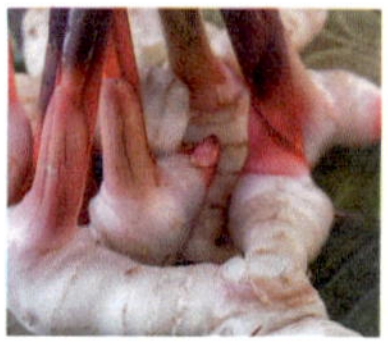

GALANGAL

Aromatic rhizomes found in Asian cooking (particularly Thai and Vietnamese), it is also used in many traditional medicines. It is thought to fight cancer and inflammation, may protect against infections, may boost male fertility, and traditional medicine has held that it aids digestion and alleviates respiratory ailments. Side effects at normal levels seem non-existent, but excessive levels seem to cause a drop in energy, diarrhea, and more.

G

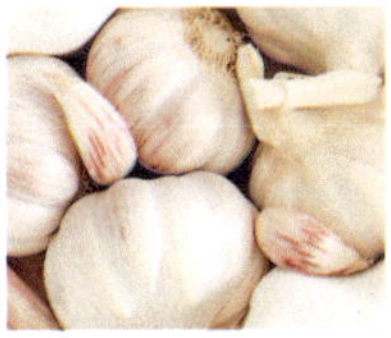

GARLIC

Native to Central Asia and Iran, garlic has clearly spread across the world. A staple of many cuisines over the past many thousands of years, garlic has been a food flavoring and used in traditional medicine. It's strong in vitamins B6 and C, and also in a lot of minerals. It is possibly effective for many ailments, such as reducing the hardening of arteries, blood pressure, and cholesterol.

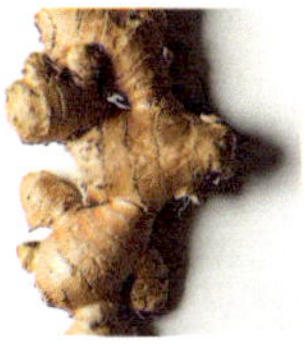

GINGER

A rhizome often used as a spice and in traditional medicine and is high in vitamin B6, magnesium, and manganese. Used for various effects in both sweet and savory foods, it also has been shown to reduce nausea due to motion sickness, chemotherapy, and pregnancy. There is also evidence it can act as an anti-inflammatory and improve digestive function.

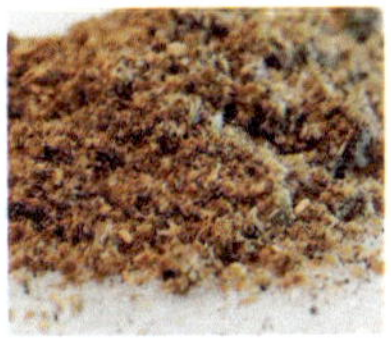

GRAM FLOUR

Not to be confused with Graham flour, this is made from the gram chickpea. It is widely used across the Indian subcontinent and has made its way to northern Africa (there is a similar flour made of garbanzo beans also used in southern Europe). It is high in folate, magnesium, phosphorus, iron, and zinc. Also, as it is not wheat, it is a good flour for those with gluten sensitivities.

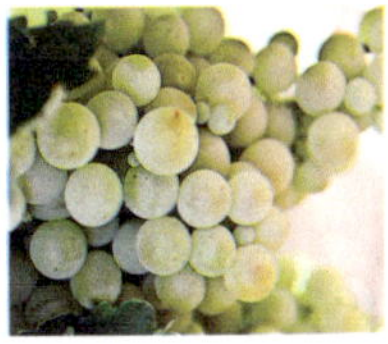

GRAPES

Grapes have been with us up to 8,000 years. Nutritionally, grapes have a decent amount of vitamin K, but not much else. However, grapes bring more than just nutrition by way of phytochemicals, and may be beneficial for the heart, circulation, eyes, and skin, and possibly work as anti-cancer agents. There are very few warnings for grapes in humans, but they are highly toxic to dogs and can lead to renal failure.

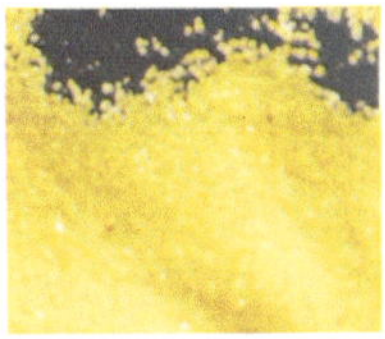

GRITS

(See Corn)

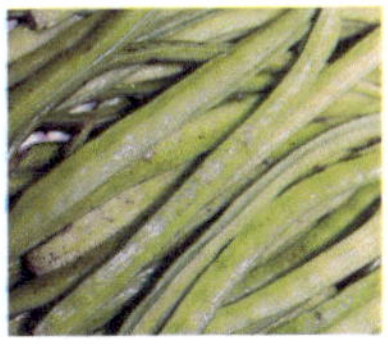

GUAR

Also known as the cluster bean. It is strong in vitamin C and iron (for those suffering from anemia, cluster beans can help quite a bit). Guar gum is also made of this, and it has five times the thickening power than corn starch. Because guar can absorb water to an extreme limit (with a bean able to swell up to 20 times its size), it can cause intestinal blockages if consumed regularly.

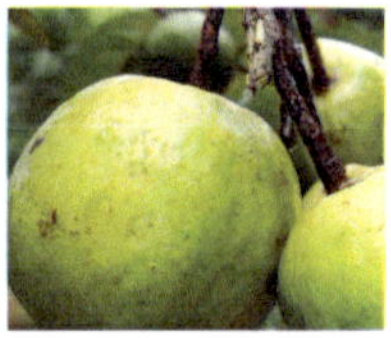

GUAVA

A tropical fruit eaten across the world, guava can be found in many cuisines. They're rich in dietary fiber, very high in vitamin C, and moderate in folate. They have been used in traditional medicine to reduce diarrhea and menstrual cramps, and research shows regular consumption can help reduce high blood pressure and possibly knee pain. Guava might lower blood sugar, so those with diabetes must take caution with it.

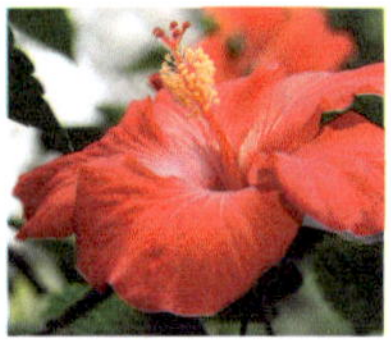

HIBISCUS

Usually red, with a tart, unique flavor, and high in vitamin C, beverages made of the flower's leaves is served in many places across the planet. The roselle is used as a vegetable in some places, and, in the Philippines, hibiscus is used as a souring agent and an ingredient in chicken soup. It can help lower blood pressure, but also can stimulate menstruation and uterine contractions, meaning it can cause an abortion in pregnant women.

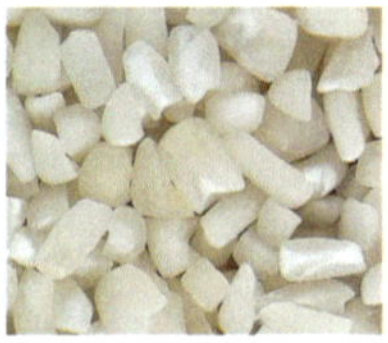

HOMINY

(See Corn)

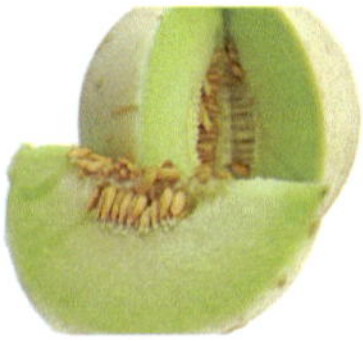

HONEYDEW

Technically a gourd and part of the muskmelon family, honeydew is usually known as an innocuous, inoffensive fruit just sitting and taking up space in a salad or on the side of a plate as a garnish. However, it contains some fat and protein, and a lot of vitamin C. It's also not considered to have a lot of side effects, meaning it can be consumed by most people with no issue. It also contains potassium, yet is low in calories.

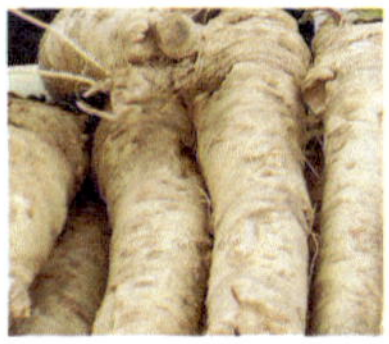

HORSERADISH

A root vegetable from the same family as mustard, broccoli, and wasabi, this is usually used as a flavoring agent and condiment in various cuisines. Horseradish contains some minerals, but is healthy for its glucosinolates, which may have health benefits in fighting bacteria and stopping spasms. It is said to help the respiratory tract, gout, colic, and intestinal worms in children.

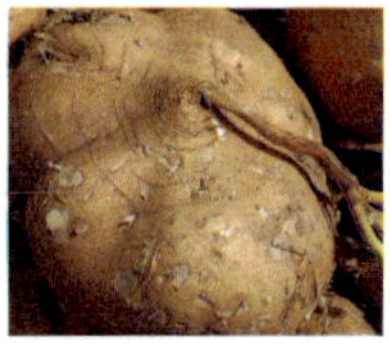

JICAMA

The root of a vine native to Mexico, it resembles a raw potato or a pear. Spaniards spread the plant to Asia, where it made its way into Filipino, Chinese, and Japanese cuisines. Moderately nutritious (only really missing sodium from the main vitamins and minerals), but high in vitamin C and rich in dietary fiber. Only the root is edible—the rest is toxic (the seeds were once used as an insecticide).

K

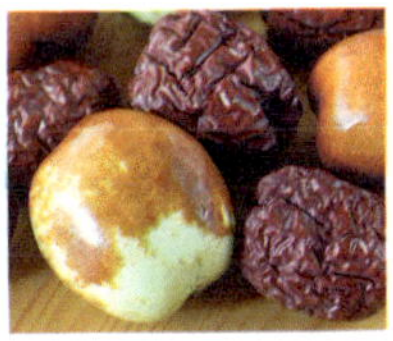

JUJUBE

The shrub bears a small, edible drupe that was domesticated in Asia over 11,000 years ago and has spread over that continent and into Europe and Africa. When fresh, the drupe is a very rich source of vitamin C, but when dried, it is very rich in vitamin B2 and an excellent source for vitamins B1 and C, and iron, magnesium, manganese, phosphorus, and potassium. In traditional medicine it is used to alleviate stress.

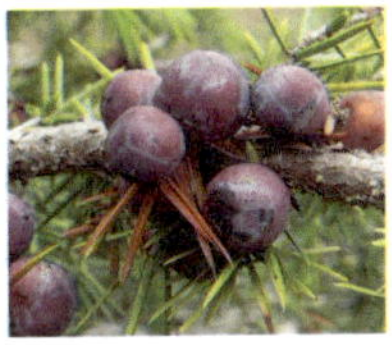

JUNIPER BERRY

The juniper berry isn't a berry—it's a seed cone of the juniper bush—and is widely used as a spice (it may be the only spice that is cultivated from conifers). They contain antioxidants and have antibacterial and antifungal properties. They may improve sleep and digestion, too. In traditional medicine, they were used as birth control, and there is a risk of miscarriage when consuming them (even in small doses).

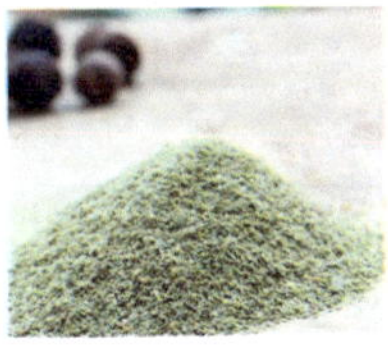

KAFFIR LIME

(See Makrut Lime)

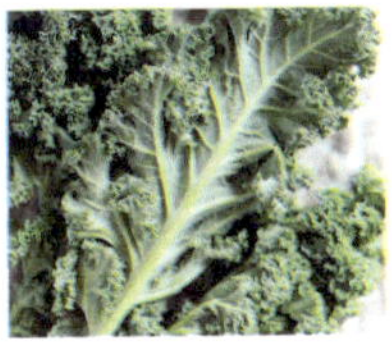

KALE

Its nutritional value is huge, with its raw state being massively rich in vitamins C and K, and being an excellent source of vitamin A equivalents, vitamins B1, B2, B5, B6, E, and folate, and also rich in calcium, iron, magnesium, manganese, phosphorus, and potassium. In addition, it is full of beneficial phytochemicals. Boiling reduces the benefits by quite a bit, but steaming, microwaving, or stir frying do not. No real side effects, but it can cause tummy troubles if you eat too much.

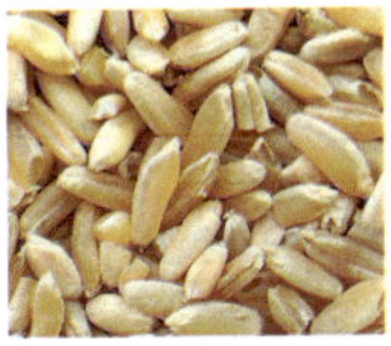

KAMUT

Kamut's grain is twice the size of modern wheat. Massively rich in vitamins B1, B3, and B6, and iron, magnesium, manganese, phosphorus, and zinc, it is also a good source of vitamins B2 and B5, in addition to potassium. It also has a high protein content and an excellent amount of dietary fiber. As with any wheat, those sensitive to gluten should avoid it.

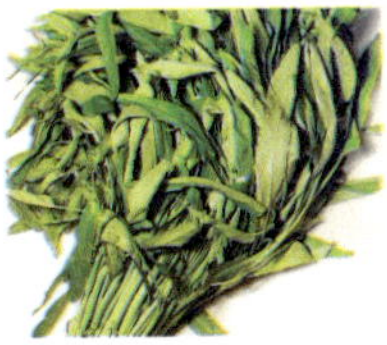

KANGKONG

Also known as "water spinach," this plant is more closely related to sweet potatoes. It is used in many Asian cuisines, including Indonesian, Thai, and Filipino. It has high levels of vitamin A equivalents, folate, vitamin C, iron, and magnesium. It has been used to treat piles, nosebleeds, and high blood pressure. There are antioxidants and anti-microbial substances, and may have a moderate anti-cancer effect.

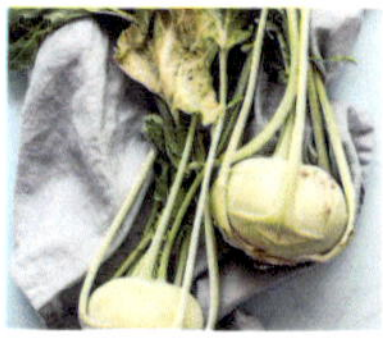

KOHLRABI

Literally German for "cabbage turnip," kohlrabi seems to have come to Europe from Asia in the 16th century. It is another member of the cabbage family and, like its cousins, is full of vitamins, minerals and fiber. It is moderately strong in most minerals and vitamins, with vitamins B6 and C being its richest sources. Some of its phytochemicals have led researchers to believe kohlrabi has antioxidants and help in preventing cancer.

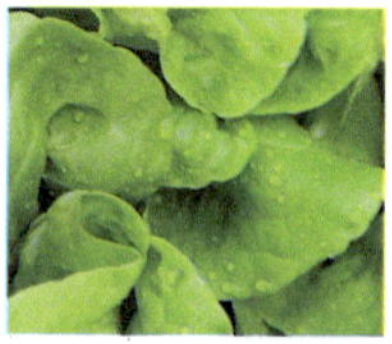

LETTUCE

Part of the daisy family, lettuce was originally farmed in ancient Egypt and spread from there. Butterhead, for example, is rich in vitamin A equivalents, beta-Carotene, folate, and iron, and it's massively rich in vitamin K. Lettuce, usually, is safe from side effects. However, as we've seen in the past few years, how the lettuce is grown can bring parasites and bacteria with it.

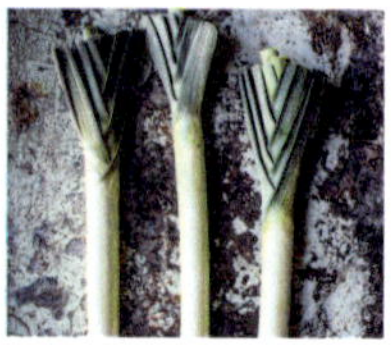

LEEK

From the same family as onions and garlic, it was first cultivated thousands of years ago. It is moderately rich in vitamin A equivalents, beta-Carotene, vitamin B6, and iron. It's very rich in vitamin K and manganese. It seems to have antioxidant, anti-cancer, and anti-inflammatory properties. For those on blood thinners or the like, the high vitamin K content can be an issue.

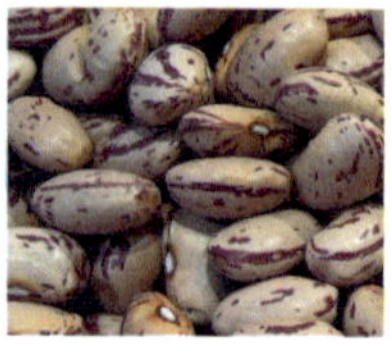

LEGUME

(See Bean, but don't necessarily say that in science class)

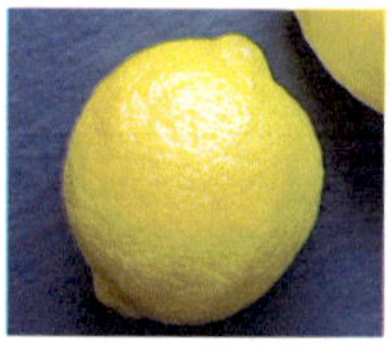

LEMON

The lemon we all know seems to a hybrid between a bitter orange and a citron. It is used in drinks, garnishes, candies, oils, and the leaves will sometimes be used in tea. Like many citrus fruits, the lemon brings a large amount of vitamin C, but not much else in terms of micronutrients. It supplies antioxidants, which, along with the citric acid, help it prevent kidney stones, improve absorption of iron, and reduce cancer risk.

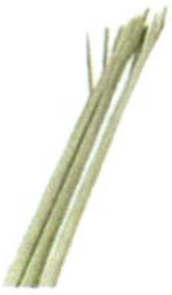

LEMONGRASS

These have been used as flavoring agents, aromatics, and for producing oils (citronella, for example) for soaps and insect repellents. It may inhibit bacteria growth and yeast, and found to control thrush in some. Traditional medicine says it reduces pain, swelling, and fever. It may improve levels of sugar and cholesterol in the blood and have antioxidant properties. It does stimulate the uterus and may start menstrual flow, so those who are pregnant should avoid it.

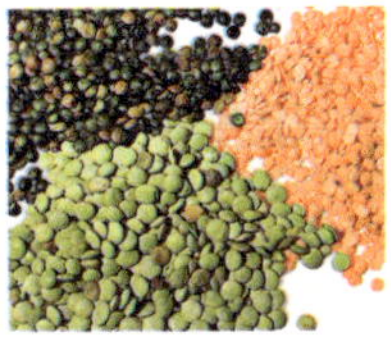

LENTIL

The oldest pulse crop known—some of the oldest specimens dating back 13,000 years ago in Greece—is it any surprise it's so well known in many cultures? Boiled lentils are a strong source of numerous nutrients, including folate, iron, manganese, magnesium, copper, zinc, and vitamin B6. The digestible starch and slowly digested starch of lentils also mean those with diabetes might find value in eating them more.

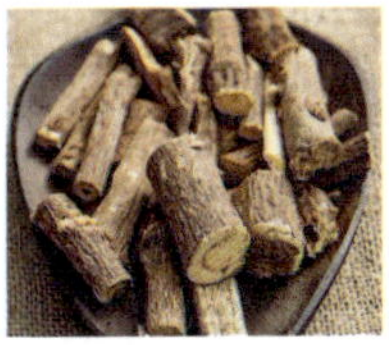

LICORICE

Not the candy—the legume! We mostly know this for the candy that shares its name (and uses its extract for the flavor and black color), but its roots in food and medicine are deep. While it is traditionally used to treat various diseases, it seems to have an effect on eczema (when applied topically) and for those who have had breathing tubes recently removed (as a lozenge).

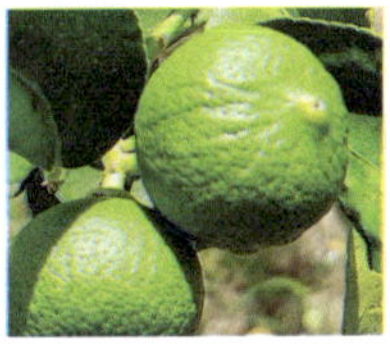

LIME

The lime originates from south and southeast Asia (South Indian cuisine is heavily based on the lime). It has a higher content of sugar and acid than lemons do, and it's used for its acidity, aroma, and pickling properties. Only vitamin C is high, but the pulp and peel bring phytochemicals with them, and those seem to help prevent stones in the kidney and gall bladder, in addition to an anti-parasite and anti-viral benefit, too.

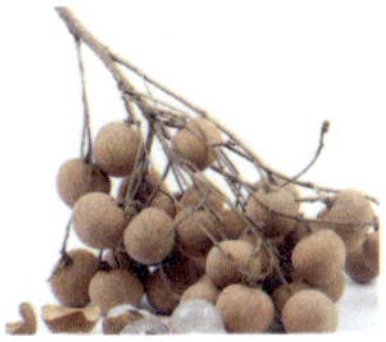

LONGAN

Its name comes from the Chinese for "dragon eye," as, when peeled, looks like an eye, the black seed staring back at you from within the translucent flesh of the fruit. It's an excellent source of vitamin C and has been shown to have anti-inflammatory properties. Traditionally, it's been used to remedy stomachache, insomnia, amnesia, and dropsy.

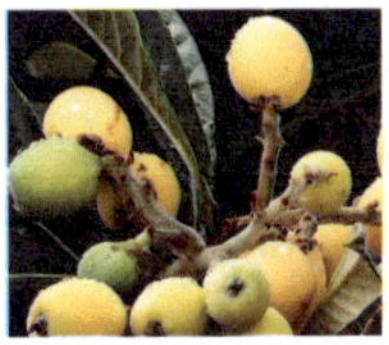

LOQUAT

Not related to kumquats (their names share an origin). The loquat is high in sugar, acid, and pectin, but low in sodium, high in vitamins A and B6, fiber, potassium, and manganese. It's eaten in various ways—juices, smoothies, canned or as part of confections (it's even used to make wine and a natural sweetener)—but very often it's eaten fresh. The seeds are toxic and should be removed when eating fresh.

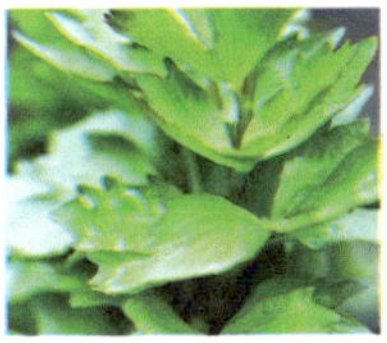

LOVAGE

Long cultivated in Europe, the leaves, roots, and seeds are used in many culinary ways. It's also used as a fragrance for soap and cosmetics. It seems to decrease spasms and, as it increases urination, it's been used to relieve various ailments of the kidneys, liver, and urinary tract. It also seems to raise blood pressure, exacerbate kidney problems, and can cause a miscarriage.

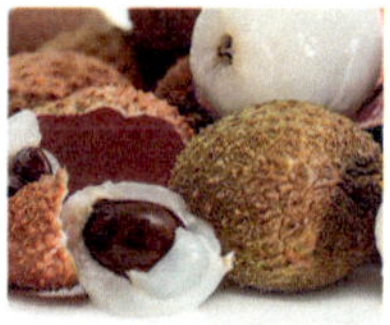

LYCHEE

The fruit of a tall evergreen tree in the tropics, it has been cultivated for over 3,000 years and typically eaten raw or in desserts. A good source of carbohydrates and a bit of protein, but it's not rich in any micronutrients other than vitamin C. It is said to be good for coughs and fever, however the seeds can cause hypoglycemia and have been linked to encephalitis outbreaks in malnourished children who ate underripe fruit.

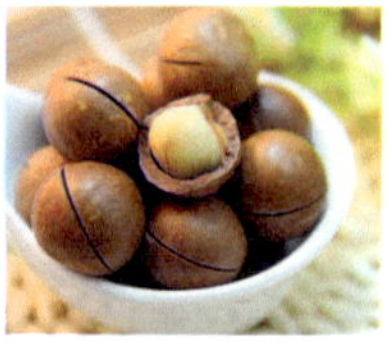

MACADAMIA

A valuable food crop. Compared to other nuts, it's high in fat and low in protein, but it is highly caloric and is a very rich source of numerous micronutrients, including vitamins B1, B2, B3, B5, and B6 in addition to iron, magnesium, manganese, phosphorus, and zinc. They are effective in helping lower cholesterol (by upwards of 9%). Those with tree nut allergies should avoid this.

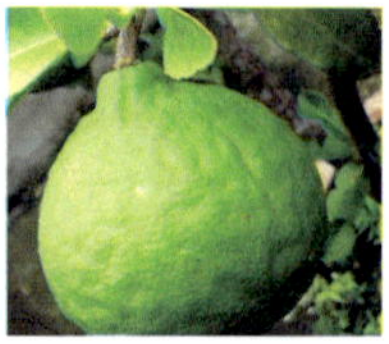

MAKRUT LIME

Do not refer to it as "kaffir" (which is a racial slur), but instead use "makrut" (as the Thai people do). The fruit, rind, and leaves are used in Thai and Cambodian cuisines (and in those across the neighboring regions). Like most citrus, it's rich in vitamin C and is a source for some folate, phosphorus, and magnesium.

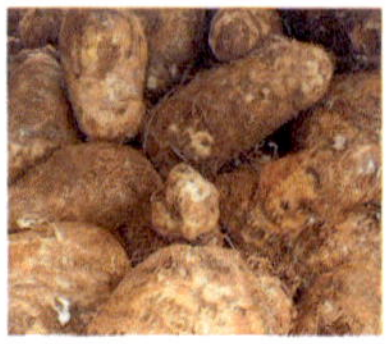

MALANGA

Sometimes mistaken for taro or eddo, it's the starchy bulbo-tuber (corm) of flowering plants from tropical America. It's described as having an earthy and nutty taste and is used in soups and stews, or grilled, fried, or puréed. The young leaves are sometimes stewed (such as callaloo). High in fiber and rich in potassium, it is also one of the least allergenic foods, and can be milled into flour.

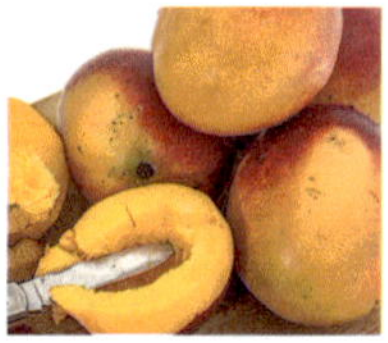

MANGO

First cultivated in south Asia thousands of years ago (where it still has deep cultural significance), it has now spread to almost every continent and tends to be used in their cuisines. It is rich in phytochemicals (that may protect against cancer and boost the immune system) and some micronutrients (vitamin C and folate, especially), but it is high in sugar. It can cause dermatitis, or even anaphylaxis, so sensitive individuals may need to stay away.

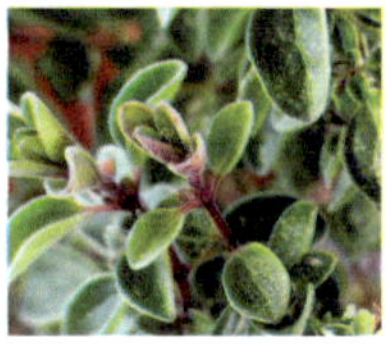

MARJORAM

In some countries it's called oregano, but they are different spices. We use the leaves (green or dry) for seasoning soups and other dishes, and in herbal teas. It has used for runny nose, cough, and cold (but can increase mucous production) and digestion issues. The oil is used as fragrance in soaps, lotions, perfumes, and cosmetics. It can start a period, so stay away when pregnant. It may slow blood clotting and heart rates.

N

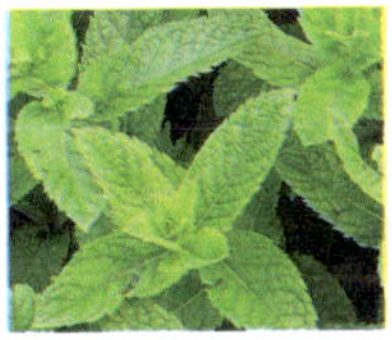

MINT

An umbrella term for a genus of plants in the mint family, this is usually referring to spearmint (but can also include both peppermint and wild mint). Mint is used heavily in cuisine, as a flavoring agent, as an aromatic, and in medicinal ways (such as using menthol to help break up congestion). It has been shown to promote brain health, remedying digestive problems, kill bacteria, and possibly fight cancerous cells.

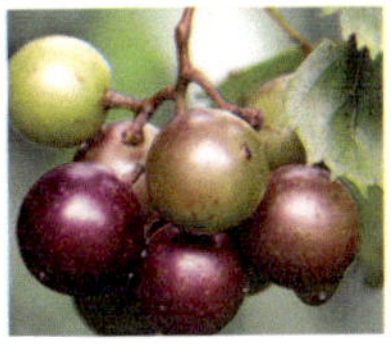

MUSCADINE GRAPE

A grape native to the United States, they are part of a separate subgenus than other grapes (and there is debate about giving them their own genus), though much of the information about grapes (including the toxicity to dogs) applies here, too. The thick, dark purple skins bring most of the benefits when eating these, as they have antioxidant and anti-inflammatory properties, are a good source of fiber.

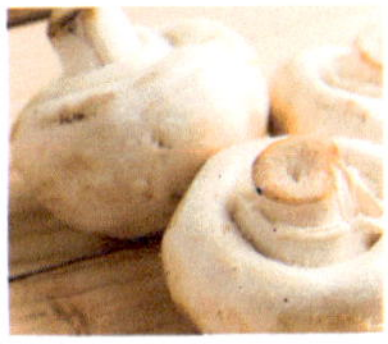

MUSHROOM

Remember, some poisonous mushrooms resemble edible ones—please don't eat any you aren't 100% sure of. In general, a mushroom is mostly water and tends to be a rich source of various B vitamins, phosphorous, potassium, selenium, and zinc. If they are exposed to UV light, they will convert it to vitamin D2. Mushrooms may boost the nervous system and have been used to treat diabetes, cancer, high cholesterol, and more.

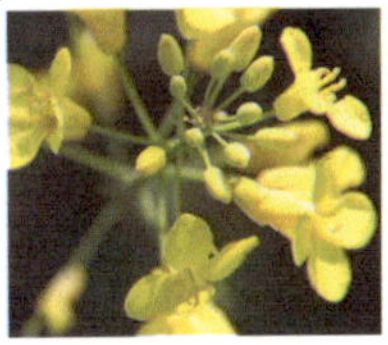

MUSTARD

Mustard comes from plants, not yellow bottles. The seeds (massive sources B and E vitamins in addition to calcium, iron, magnesium, phosphorus, potassium, and zinc) can be fried or turned into an oil (or the condiment), and the leaves (which, even cooked, are rich in vitamins C, E, K and calcium) are often served in salads and stir fries. Those with allergies to mugwort pollen, nuts, and peaches or plums should avoid.

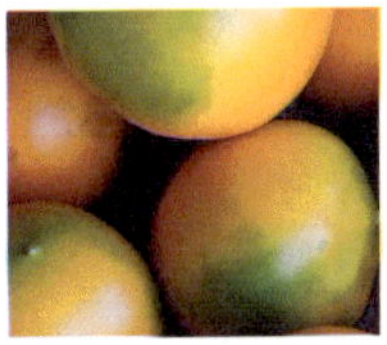

NARANJILLA

A nightshade with a moderate amount of carbohydrates, dietary fiber, iron, potassium, and vitamins B5, B6, C, and E. It's massively rich in vitamin K. It might be useful in preventing cancer, strengthening bones, bolstering the immune system. It encourages urination and may help detoxify your body. The fuzz on the outside of the fruit may irritate sensitive skin, and those allergic to nightshade should stay away.

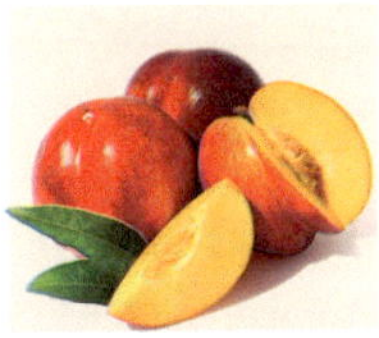

NECTARINE

(See Peach)

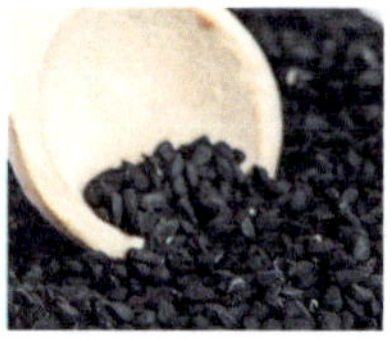

NIGELLA SATIVA

Also referred to as "black seed and "back cumin," humans have used N. sativa as a spice and flavoring going back at least 3,000 years. It is a decent source for fiber, calcium, iron, and magnesium. There is some evidence it can help lower blood pressure and reduce cholesterol, and it's been used traditionally for headaches, congestion, asthma, arthritis, and parasites. Large amounts should be avoided by pregnant women.

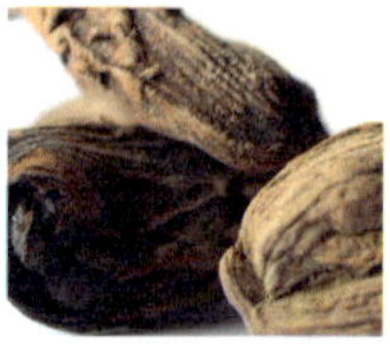

NUTMEG

This spice has been with us for at least 3,500 years. And usually used as a spice, essential oils and nutmeg butter are also made from it (along with the red covering—the spice mace—and the pericarp, which is used to make jelly). High in fiber (but not much else), it can be used to alleviate pain from cavities in baby teeth and has been used to address many other ailments.

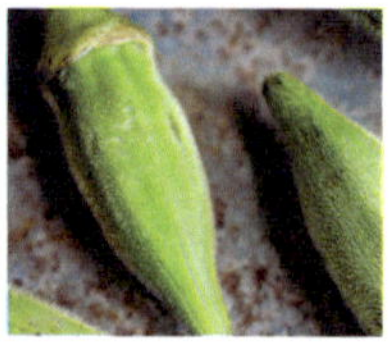

OKRA

The edible seed pods of a flowering plant in the mallow family, okra's origins are unknown, but it has become a staple of many cuisines. Rich in vitamins, magnesium, and fiber, it can improve digestion, boost the immune system, lower blood pressure, and seems to have positive effects on asthma. It is also rich in oxalates, which can bind with kidney and gallstones, making them worse. Those taking metformin should not eat okra.

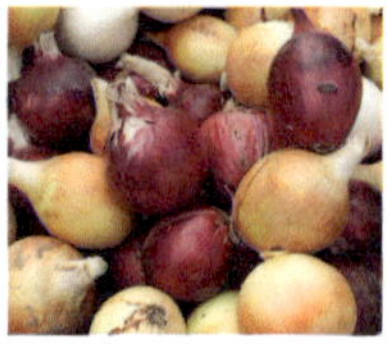

ONION

Widely cultivated, its use goes back roughly 7,000 years. European settlers brought it to North America—only to find it was already widespread! There is some evidence it can reduce blood sugar in those with diabetes and may reduce risk of stomach cancer, in addition to research showing a gel with onion extract can improve scarring.

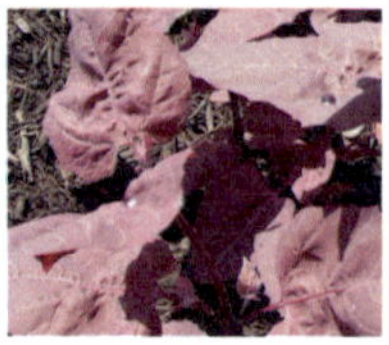

ORACHE

A hardy annual plant that was grown in the Mediterranean (until spinach became more favored) with a salty and spinach-like taste. The leaves can be cooked or used raw, and were once used to color pasta. It has been used for menstrual cramps and for starting menstrual flow (those who are pregnant should avoid it).

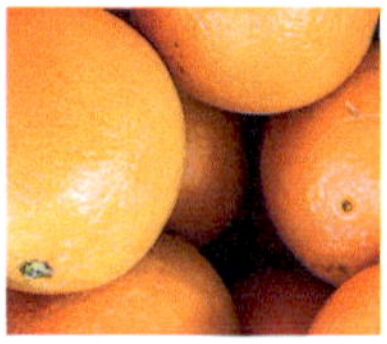

ORANGE

Orange trees are the most cultivated fruit trees in the world, they are used for their fruit, juice, and rinds, are rich in vitamin C and the pulp is a good source of fiber. The juice seems to be effective in fighting high cholesterol and high blood pressure and reducing the risk of stroke. Large amounts of the peel in children can have severe side effects, including death.

P

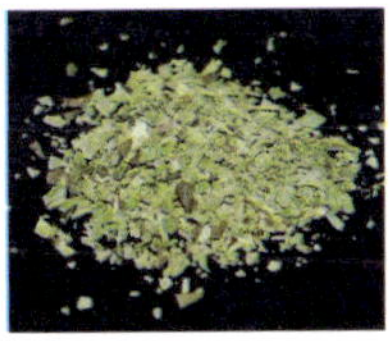

OREGANO

This is sometimes the name given to marjoram, but they are different plants. Heavily used in cuisines across the Mediterranean and Latin America. It has been shown that oregano can reduce high cholesterol kill various intestinal parasites. As oregano can lower blood sugar levels and can increase the risk of bleeding, it is best not to use oregano in medicinal amounts while pregnant.

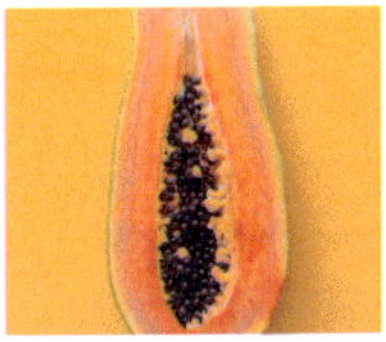

PAPAYA

Native to Latin America, the papaya has migrated across tropical regions (particularly southeast Asia) and their cuisines. It is eaten raw, cooked, and pickled in a wide variety of dishes. Rich in vitamin C and moderate in folate, but otherwise lacking significant amounts of nutrients, it's thought it may fight certain types of cancers, dengue fever, diabetes, gingivitis, and periodontitis.

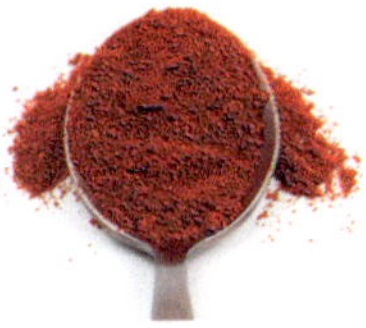

PAPRIKA

The spice made from dried and ground chili peppers from the Americas. The medicinal benefits from paprika (or any pepper-based spice or supplement) is due to capsicum, which is utilized in treating nerve pain (in diabetics) and nerve damage (from shingles), but also back pain, cluster headaches, osteoarthritis, and more. It's also very nutrient-rich, and brings a few carotenoids with it.

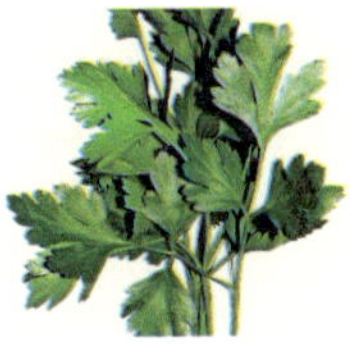

PARSLEY

That innocuous green sprig you ignore as "garnish" on your plate is amazing for you. It's so ever present in so many dishes that we tend to ignore it. It's a great source of flavonoids and antioxidants, vitamins A, C, a massive amount of K, and beta-carotene, calcium, iron, magnesium, potassium, and zinc. It can lower blood sugar, reduce blood clotting, and can also increase water retention.

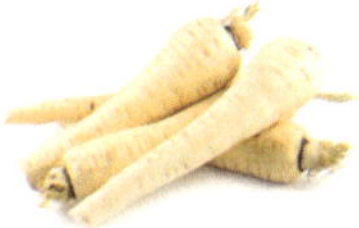

PARSNIPS

A root vegetable originally grown in Eurasia, they are usually baked, boiled, roasted, gilled, used in stews, or as a side. Rich in vitamins and minerals (which are close to the skin, so don't peel them), and a good source of fiber (helping constipation and cholesterol), and possibly has anti-cancer, anti-inflammatory, and anti-fungal properties. The plant's sap can cause phytophotodermatitis.

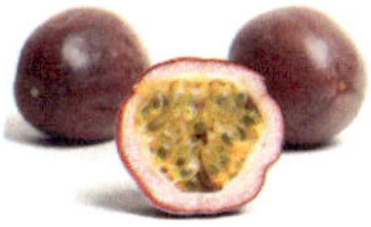

PASSION FRUIT

The fruit is different than others I've gone into here because it's not the flesh we eat—it's the seeds! It's rich in phytochemicals rich source of antioxidants, minerals, vitamins, and fiber. It may be useful in reducing the risks of diabetes, heart disease, and obesity. It is also being studied in its effects as an anti-inflammatory, relieving arthritis pain, and treating asthma.

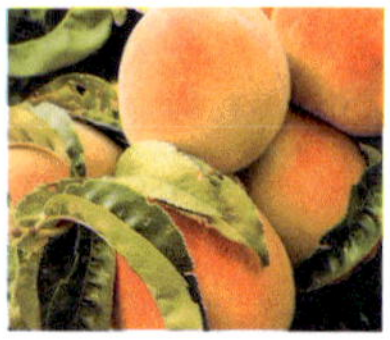

PEACH

Despite the fuzz, these and nectarines are the same species. Not very nutritious, its phytochemicals seem to help prevent cancer, act as an anti-fungal and anti-inflammatory, combat anemia, and help the cardiovascular system. There are peach allergies, but usually peeled and canned fruit can be tolerated. The pits can create the toxic cyanide gas, and there is a link of colorectal cancer in men if overconsumed.

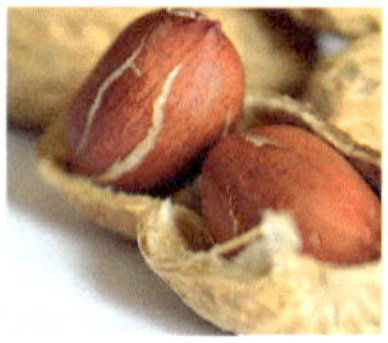

PEANUT

We have all learned about peanut allergies, but the peanut is still a versatile and useful crop for many across the globe. Whole, as an oil, butter, or flour (gluten-free), this legume is packed with vitamins (no C, though), minerals, proteins, fats, fiber, and phytochemicals. Evidence is pointing to eating nuts daily, including peanuts, can help reduce the risk of heart disease.

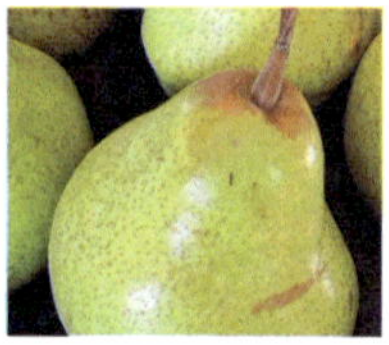

PEAR

These have been with us since prehistoric times. The ancient Romans and Chinese both ate pears, and many languages use similar words for its name. Is it any surprise 23.7 million tons were produced in 2018? As tasty and ubiquitous as they are, they aren't overly nutritious (though they are a moderate source of fiber), but there are also few-to-no side effects.

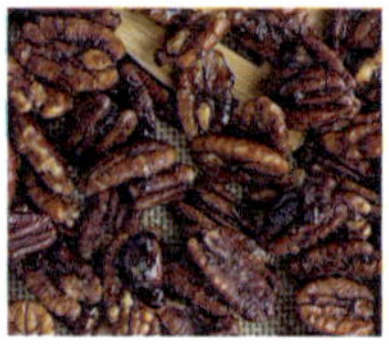

PECAN

Native to the southern region of the USA. Despite being part of some caloric treats, it is a rich source of fat, protein, fiber, and plenty of vitamins and minerals. They seem to improve cardiovascular health, brain function, metabolism, and may lower cholesterol and cancer risk. There can be allergic reactions, but most are able to eat them without issue (assuming you don't eat an entire vegan pecan pie at once).

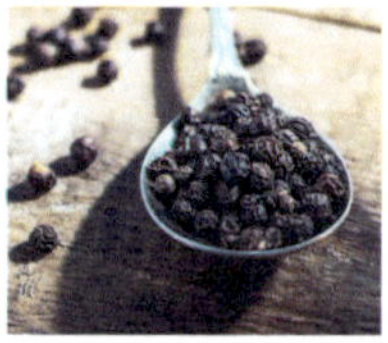

PEPPERCORN

(See Black Pepper)

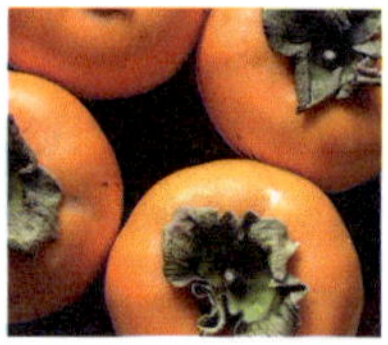

PERSIMMON

Native to Japan, China, and Korea. They are eaten fresh, dried, or cooked, and are used in various desserts and beverages. A good source of dietary fiber and manganese, but not rich in any other micronutrients. It may lower cholesterol, and the leaf extract may lower blood sugar in those with prediabetes. It may cause allergies, and like any food with a high fiber content, eating a lot may result in GI blockages.

P

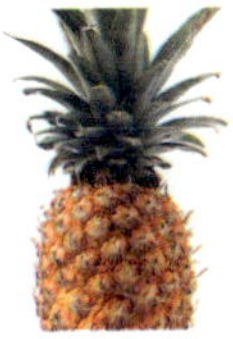

PINEAPPLE

It originated in South America, making its way to Central America, and later spread by the Spanish. Heavily used around the world, it is commonplace as raw fruit, juice, in desserts, in alcoholic beverages, or even a pizza topping. Very rich in vitamin C and manganese, it also brings a group of enzymes called bromelain, which seems to ease skin conditions, joint swelling, knee pain, and ulcerative colitis.

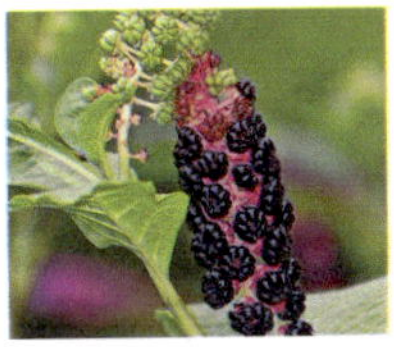

POKEWEED

All parts of the plant are poisonous (a single berry can kill a child) and it should only be handled by those who know what they are doing with it. The leaves and stems of young plants can be eaten, but must be boiled twice (at least). It's rich in vitamins A, B2, C, and K, and fairly rich in manganese. Native Americans and early settlers used it to treat joint pain, mumps, tonsilitis, cancers, and skin infections.

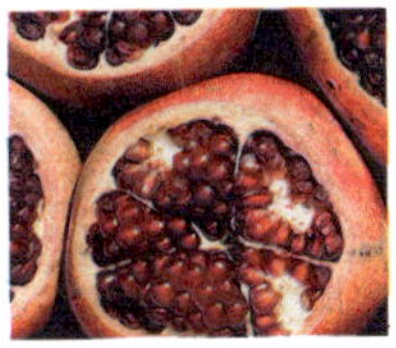

POMEGRANATE

Cultivated since ancient times in the Mediterranean, it has spread to many regions around the world (and their cuisines). It has been used raw, as juice, as part of dessert, as wine, sauce, and even a spice (anar dana). It is a good source of vitamins C, K, and folate, and a very good source of fiber. The root, stem, and peel contain poisons and should not be ingested (though peel extracts are used as dietary supplements).

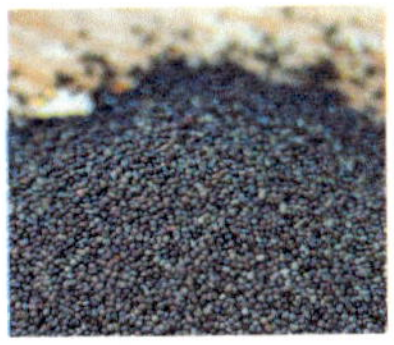

POPPY SEED

Used in a great number of cuisines in cakes and curries and more, poppy seeds are a rich source of fiber, vitamins B1, B6, E, and folate, iron, magnesium, manganese, phosphorus, and zinc. They have been used to ease asthma, constipation, and insomnia. Oh, and the witch knew what she was doing when she put Dorothy and friends to sleep in the poppy field—they contain morphine.

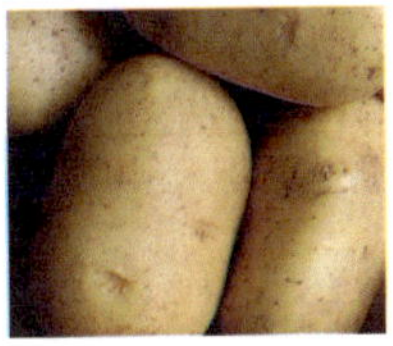

POTATO

Native to the Americas, the potato has become the world's fourth-largest food crop. Prepared in ways too numerous to list here, it is almost ubiquitous at meals in many parts of the world. Drinking potato juice improves the feeling of indigestion in some, and purple potatoes seem to reduce stiffness in the arteries and reduce blood pressure levels. Avoid if you are on a low glycemic index diet.

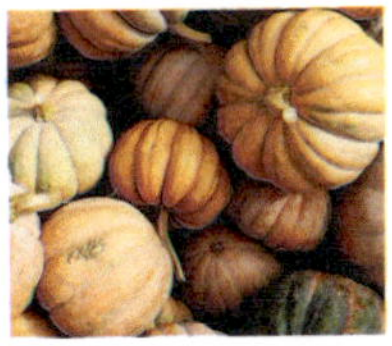

PUMPKIN

Very versatile in their cooking uses, from soup to pie to roasted seeds, they are a good source of vitamins A and C and beta-carotene. Traditional medicine holds it's a good treatment for urinary ailments and intestinal worms, and there is research backing those up. Pumpkin also seems to be further beneficial to men specifically, as it has been shown to have effects on male pattern baldness and enlarged prostates.

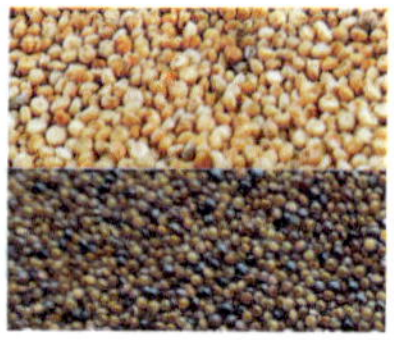

QUINOA

Humans first ate this 4,000 years ago in South America, and now more than 70 countries produce—should that really be a surprise? It's not a grass, but rather a gluten-free seed rich in protein, fiber, B vitamins, and many minerals. It can be used to make flour, soup, and even beer. It seems to make us feel more full than wheat or rice, and may decrease triglycerides.

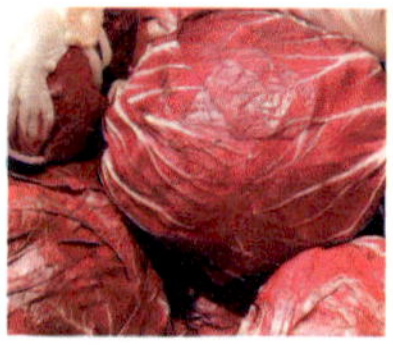

RADICCHIO

A chicory popular in Italian cuisines, and is usually grilled or roasted or used as a topping or a side. It's not overly rich in minerals, but is very strong in antioxidants, vitamin K and moderately strong in folate and vitamins C and E. It was said that using it in coffee for too long would damage the eyes, but there is no evidence to support that.

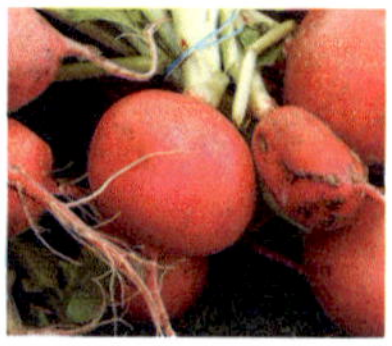

RADISH

Originally domesticated in Asia, it's now present in many cuisines. It supplies a decent amount of vitamin C and a smattering of other micronutrients. It has been used for disorders of the GI tract, liver, and more. It's also used to reduce high cholesterol. It can lower blood sugar and increase bile flow (which can increase pain if a gallstone is blocking the bile duct). Large amounts can irritate the GI tract.

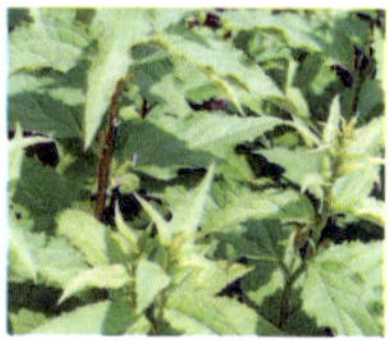

RAMPION

A flowering biennial, it has an edible root that looks like a small turnip. In Queen Elizabeth I's time, rampion was quite popular in England (especially in winter salads), but no more. It can still be found, however, and the leaves are strong in vitamin C. It's said to be good for inflammation of the mouth and throat. An Italian tradition claims rampion makes children quarrel, however, so maybe you shouldn't leave it near the kids.

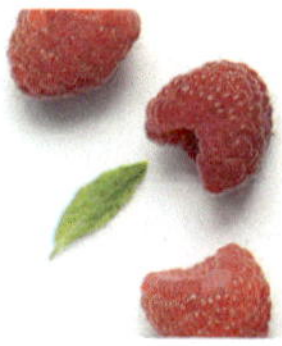

RASPBERRY

The raspberry seems to have been with us since paleolithic times, and they were associated with fertility in Greek myth. Rich in vitamin C and manganese, there's a decent amount of fiber found in them, too. The berries contain quite a few phytochemicals that are being studied to see if they are beneficial to humans. The leaf and the berry can act like estrogen, so it's best not to take the leaf during pregnancy.

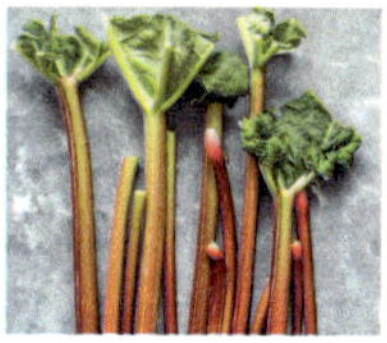

RHUBARB

Used for thousands of years in traditional Chinese medicine, the culinary rhubarb seems to have originated in Europe. The stalk is now used in pies, crumbles, and even as a treat. Traditional Chinese medicine it could be used as a laxative (no research backs that up), but is has been found to be effective with canker and cold sores, and easing the effects of menopause and pancreatitis.

S

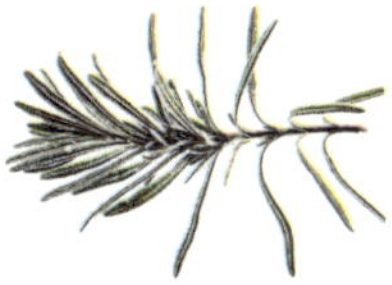

ROSEMARY

The first mentions of this herb date back 7,000 years, and it slowly made its way across the world. It's easy to grow, drought-resistant, and attractive, which explains why it has become so readily available. In a regular amount, it gives almost no nutritional value, but its extract can improve the shelf life of omega 3-rich oils. Rosemary, both by mouth and in aromatherapy, is shown to improve memory.

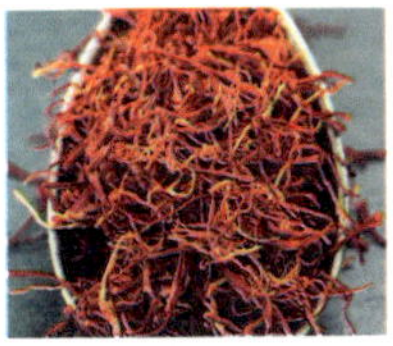

SAFFRON

We don't often think of the spice trade now, but due to the labor necessary to harvest it, saffron is an excellent example of that trade in the modern day (a kilogram can cost $5,000). It is used in cuisines across Europe and Asia, and as a dye, fragrance, and medicine. Nutritionally, it's only rich in manganese, but chemically it can alter moods, kill cancer, decrease swelling, and act like an antioxidant.

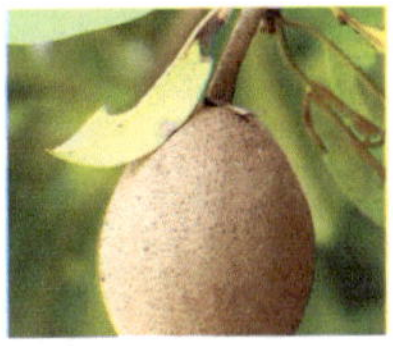

SAPODILLA

A berry from a slow-growing evergreen native to Latin America that is high in calories, fiber, and vitamin C. The fruit can be harvested twice a year (and flowering may happen year round). It tastes like a pear and is often used in desserts. The leaves have shown anti-diabetic, antioxidant, and cholesterol-lowering effects. The seeds are hooked, so it's advisable not to swallow them, and eating the raw fruit can cause difficulty breathing.

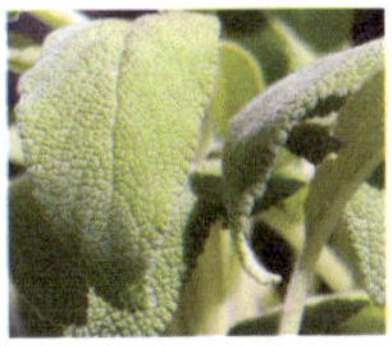

SAGE

Considered an "essential herb" in Britain, sage is heavily used in European and American cooking. It is also used to flavor tea in the Middle East. Traditional medicine holds that it helps reduce hot flashes, and may aid in digestion. Some research suggests sage has a positive influence on memory—including those suffering from Alzheimer's—and may help those who suffer from Type II diabetes.

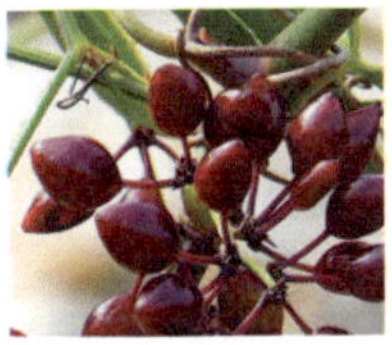

SARSAPARILLA

This is properly known as Smilax ornate, a trailing vine native to Central America and is, indeed, used to create a soft drink called "sarsaparilla, which isn't root beer (that originally came from this and sassafras, which has been found to be carcinogenic). It was considered to have medicinal properties by Native Americans and was used as a syphilis treatment.

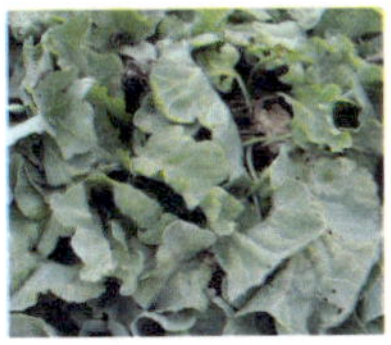

SEA KALE

A kale-looking plant growing along Europe's coasts, it's is not as nutritious (though it hasn't been studied as much). Rich in vitamin C, it seems to have anti-cancer and anti-fungal properties. The leaves have been used to heal wounds and the seeds' juice has been used to treat GI ailments. Young leaves are eaten like spinach, the shoots cooked like asparagus. The young flower buds and roots can also be consumed.

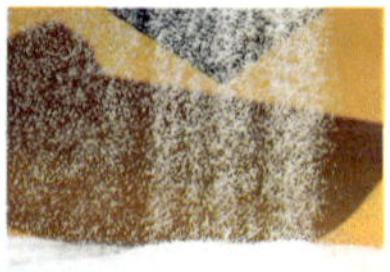

SEMOLINA

Purified wheat middlings of durum wheat used to make couscous and pasta. It's used in numerous dishes, sweet and savory, across the United States, Europe, Africa, and the Middle East. Rich in vitamins B1, B2, and folate, it's also a good source of iron, magnesium, phosphorus, and zinc. Those who are sensitive to gluten, have celiac disease, or a wheat allergy should stay away.

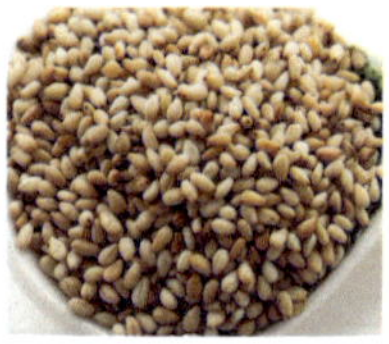

SESAME

One of the oldest oilseed crops, sesame has become commonplace in numerous cuisines. Despite its ubiquity and its regular presence, we shouldn't ignore it as it's rich in carbohydrates, dietary fiber, B vitamins, calcium, iron, magnesium, phosphorus, and zinc. It can trigger allergic reactions and be a source of allergy-triggering proteins. Cross-reactivity with other food allergens exists, too.

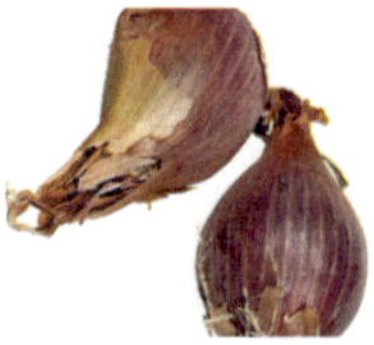

SHALLOT

(See Onion)

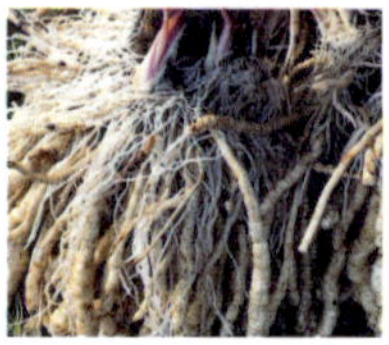

SKIRRET

Similar to the parsnip and black salsify, little nutrition data exists for it, but it is thought help with digestion and constipation when boiled and the roots seem to be rich in minerals. It has been used in various sweet and savory pies and fritters. As there has been little studied of it, it's difficult to say who may be allergic, so tread carefully if you have any conditions or allergies.

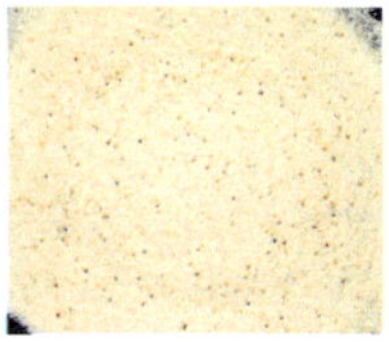

SOOJI

(See Semolina)

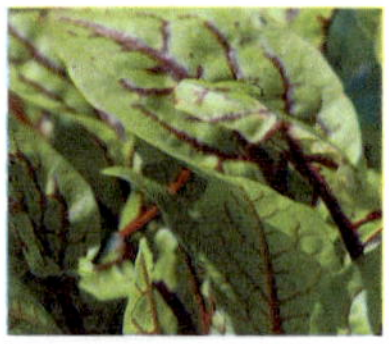

SORREL

A perennial cultivated as an herb or a salad vegetable and used in numerous preparations of soups and curries (and battered and deep fried in Afghanistan). It has a decent amount of dietary fiber, is strong in vitamins A and C, and copper, iron, magnesium, and manganese. Its sour taste comes from oxalic acid, that can be toxic and also could increase the risk of kidney disease.

S

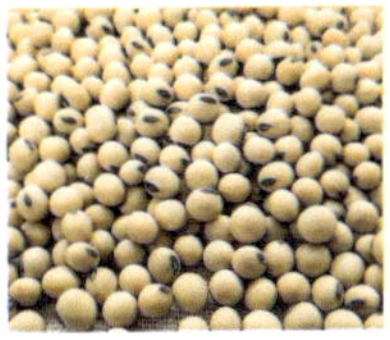

SOYBEAN

The soybean has given us tofu, natto, tempeh, and much more. Its products are exceptional sources of carbohydrates, fat, protein, and essential vitamins and minerals, and offer a lot of benefits against disease. Soy may adversely affect cystic fibrosis, various existing cancers, hypothyroidism, kidney ailments, and diabetes. Children with milk allergies may also be allergic to soy.

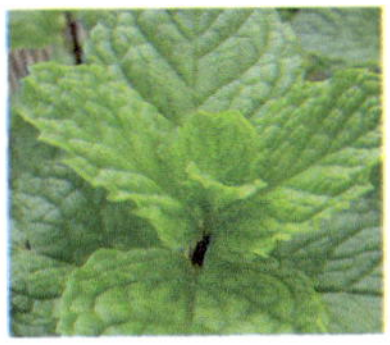

SPEARMINT

(See Mint)

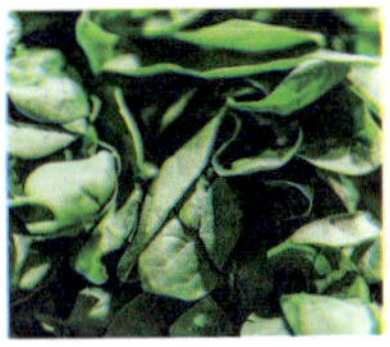

SPINACH

For all its benefits, it works against its own iron and calcium, as it also has oxalates, which render the iron unusable and decrease the absorption of calcium. Regardless, it's still strong in vitamins A, C, and K, magnesium, manganese, and folate. Those taking blood thinners, with diabetes, with latex, chard, or beet allergies, or with kidney disease need to avoid.

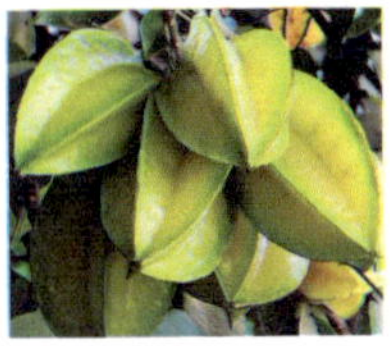

STARFRUIT

When looked at from the end, the carambola looks like a star with five points—hence the name. Popular in tropical regions, it is eaten in savory and sweet dishes, as a seasoning, and juiced. Its low calorie content and fiber make up for its lack of micronutrients (vitamin C being the major one). It may also be an anti-inflammatory and an anti-cancer agent.

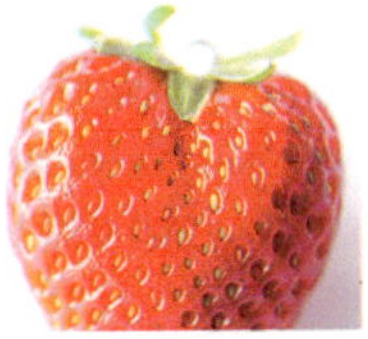

STRAWBERRY

The strawberry is a great source of vitamin C and manganese (and does supply many other nutrients—just not at large levels). However, its phytochemicals tell another story—it contains antioxidants and seems to work as an anti-cancer agent. It may also slow down how fast the nervous system ages, which might help prevent Alzheimer's and other diseases of the nervous system. It may slow blood clotting.

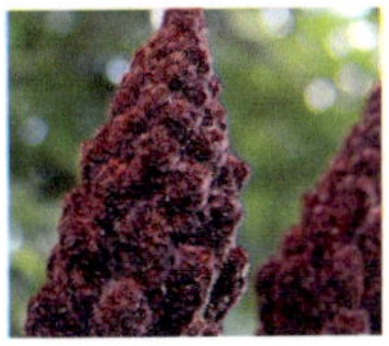

SUMAC

Don't confuse sweet sumac (red drupes) with poison sumac (white drupes)—poison sumac is, as it says, poisonous. The spice you can get from sweet sumac brings almost no nutrients with it. Instead, it's a packed full of phytochemicals that pack antioxidants and bring the ability to affect blood sugar, reduce cholesterol, reduce bone loss, and may relieve muscle pain. Furthermore, no real side effects have been discovered as of yet.

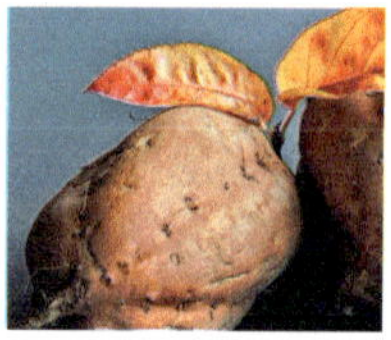

SWEET POTATO

This is not a yam. Its nutritional value has been ranked highest against other foods, as it is rich in complex carbohydrates, fiber, beta-carotene, manganese, and vitamins B5 and B6. It may benefit those suffering from diabetes and cancer, and it might reduce inflammation and boost your immune system. Avoid if you have heart or kidney disease.

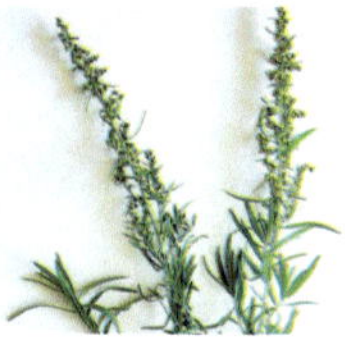

TARRAGON

Sometimes called "mugwort," but it's not that plant, it is an herb used as a spice in the kitchen (avoid Russian tarragon as it's weaker in flavor, as a fragrance in cosmetics and soaps, and in a popular soft drink in parts of the former Soviet Union. It's a good source of potassium, and it may be an anti-fungal. It may slow blood clotting. If you have allergies to ragweed, daisies, marigolds, and many others, avoid this.

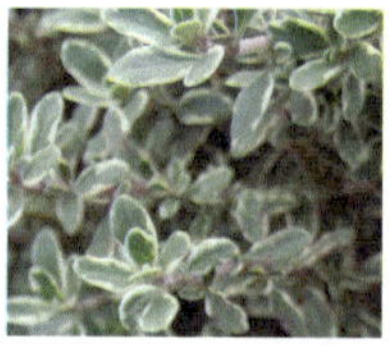

THYME

The ancient Egyptians used it as part of their embalming. The Greeks used it in baths and burnt it in their temples. Now it's sold fresh and dried, and used in either leaf form or sprig form. It has been used to ease various ailments in the past, but it seems to have antibacterial and antifungal properties, might soothe spasms (like coughing), and have antioxidant effects.

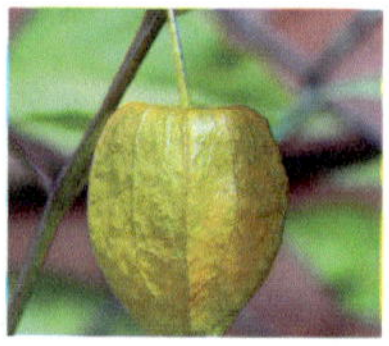

TOMATILLO

While a nightshade and looking a bit like a tomato, they aren't tomatoes. If you're familiar with Latin American cuisines, you've likely had it (salsa verde, anyone?). They're a good source of vitamins A and C, and potassium (other micronutrients are present, but not in large amounts). They seem to improve arthritis symptoms, may help reduce cancer risk, and prevent vision loss.

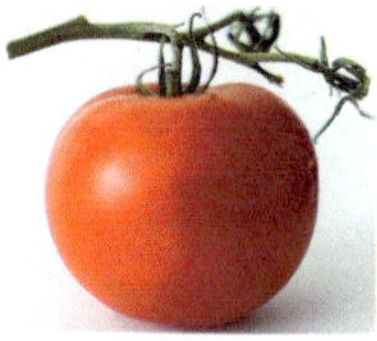

TOMATO

It is a moderate source of vitamin C and supplies other micronutrients in lesser amounts. Culinarily, the tomato brings an umami flavor. It is also possible its lycopene can assist DNA, UV-damaged skin, heart function, and vision (it's better to get the lycopene from tomato juice or paste). In large amounts, the leaves and unripe tomatoes can be toxic, and those with nightshade allergies should avoid.

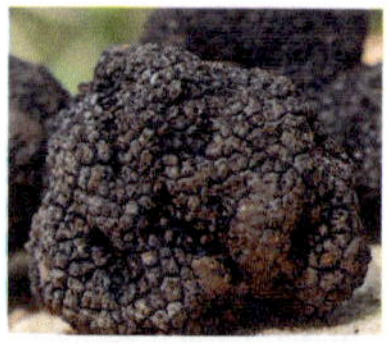

TRUFFLE

(See Mushroom)

W-Y

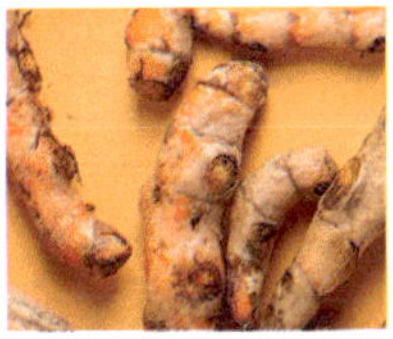

TURMERIC

A spice with a warm flavor, its curcumin is being researched. It may reduce hay fever, depression, cholesterol, itching in those with kidney disease, and osteoarthritis pain. It can slow blood clotting, block iron absorption, and can make liver disease, gallbladder problems, and estrogen-sensitive diseases worse. It may also interfere with the body's response to COVID-19, so avoid if you've been exposed.

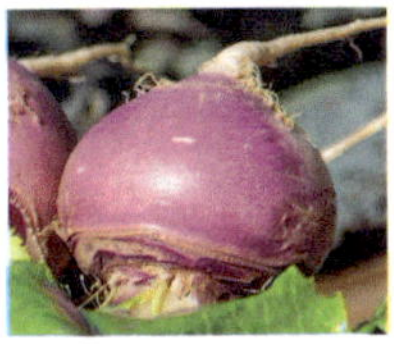

TURNIP

A root vegetable related to mustards and radishes, the greens are very nutritious as they are rich in many vitamins (lacking in the B vitamins except B6 and folate), calcium, and manganese. The roots have small amounts of all the micronutrients, except a moderate amount of vitamin C, but have anti-cancer and anti-inflammatory properties, and may help digestion, metabolism, and in losing weight.

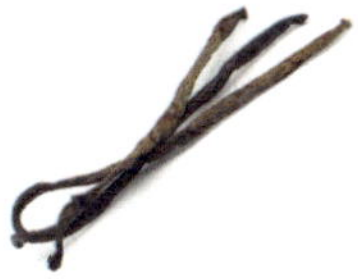

VANILLA

A relatively recent plant to be domesticated, its origins are in Mexico in the 15th century. Of course, it's used as a seasoning, a flavoring agent, in aromatics, and as a fragrance. While there is little research to back it up, it is also said to be an antibacterial, anti-depressant, pain reliever that has anti-aging and anti-cancer benefits, and seems to be good at fighting nausea. The sap of the orchid can cause a contact dermatitis.

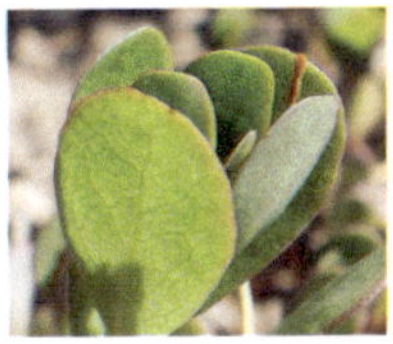

WATER PURSLANE

(See Brooklime)

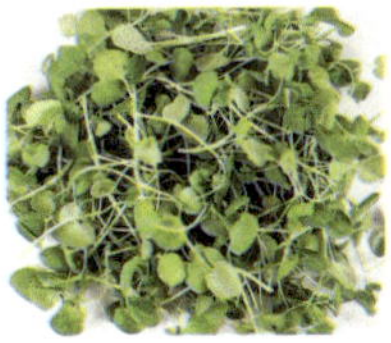

WATERCRESS

One of the oldest known leaf vegetables. Quite rich in vitamins (A, B2, B6, C, and an overabundance of K), it also has quite a bit of calcium and manganese. It's been claimed to reduce inflammation of the airways, flu, arthritis, baldness, and even constipation—but there is research showing watercress may be able to block some carcinogens and can increase the amount of urine produced by the body.

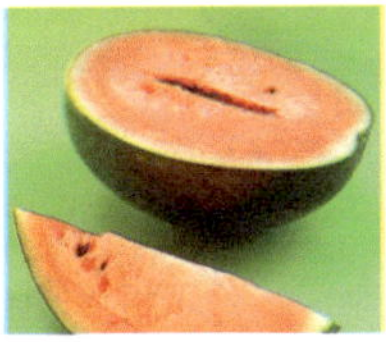

WATERMELON

At 91% water, it doesn't have a lot of micronutrients (mostly vitamin C), but does has a low glycemic load, and is just tasty. Eaten raw, juiced, or cooked, it's a versatile food. It's high in lycopene (more than 30 mg per day of which can cause tummy trouble), which may help prevent various cancers and reduce the risk of heart disease. If you are on a low carbohydrate, renal, or low potassium diet, you should avoid it.

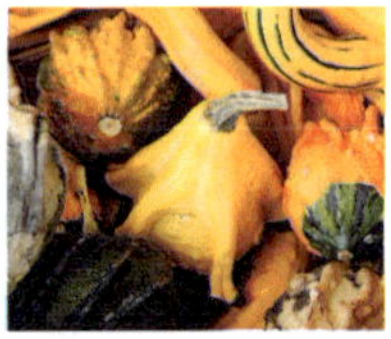

WINTER SQUASH

An umbrella term for species that have hardened rinds and can be stored for winter. In general, these are full of complex carbohydrates, fiber, vitamins A and C, potassium, and manganese. They're also decent sources of folate, vitamins B1, B3, B5, and B6. Spaghetti squash is an exception, as it's lower in fiber and vitamins than the others, but it's also lower in calories and carbohydrates.

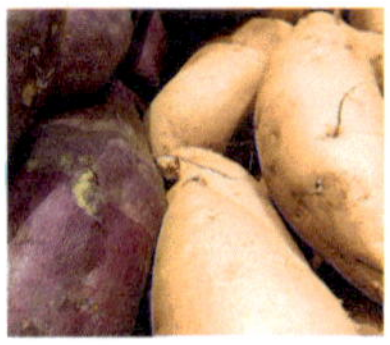

YAM

This is not a sweet potato, but is a potato crop (with a lower glycemic index). It has a decent amount of fiber, potassium, manganese, and vitamins B1, B6, and C. Wild yams may be used as an alternative to estrogen therapy for menopause or menstrual problems and, while it may not affect a pregnancy, diseases that are estrogen sensitive could be affected adversely. Those with protein S deficiency should avoid.

ACKNOWLEDGMENTS & CREDITS

I would like to thank my husband and family.
Geoffrey Sperl for editing and consultation.
Quileen Adams for design and photography.
People for the Ethical Treatment of Animals (PETA).
And various planters, photographers and artists including:

Textile Napkin, page 63.
Sheila Melissa Palmer of Quetarshe Historical
& Contemporary Textiles
www.QuetarsheTextiles.com

Anasazi, page 94 - Nomadic Lass
Havre, MT USA.
https://commons.wikimedia.org/wiki/File:Anasazi_beans_(11002990623).jpg
(Cropped & color edits)

Anise seed, page 92 - OttawaAC
https://commons.wikimedia.org/wiki/File:Anise_Seed.jpg (Cropped & color edits)

Asafoetida, page 93 - Doug Beckers
www.flickr.com/photos/dougbeckers/3756144334
(Cropped & color edits)

Atemoya, page 93 - Webysther Nunes
https://commons.wikimedia.org/wiki/File:Webysther_20150411131320_-_Atemoya.jpg
(Cropped & color edits)

Burdock root, page 96
National Institute of Korean Language
https://commons.wikimedia.org/wiki/File:Burdock_root_2.jpg (Cropped & color edits)

Cardoon, page 97 - Alexandra Carter
www.flickr.com/photos/lidfotos/15789488097
(Cropped & color edits)

Jujube, page 106 - Jacqueline Gabardy
https://commons.wikimedia.org/wiki/File:Jujube_fruit.jpg (Cropped & color edits)

Chufa, page 100 - Marco Schmidt
https://commons.wikimedia.org/wiki/File:Cyperus_esculentus_MS_4388.jpg
(Cropped & color edits)

Endive, page 102 - David Monniaux
https://commons.wikimedia.org/wiki/File:Endive_p1160063.jpg
(Cropped & color edits)

Horseradish, page 105 - Amanda Slater
Coventry, West Midlands, UK.
https://commons.wikimedia.org/wiki/File:Hren_(Horseradish)_(25955939202).jpg
(Cropped & color edits)

Jicama, page 105 - Eric in SF
https://commons.wikimedia.org/wiki/File:Pachyrhizus_erosus_2.jpg (Cropped & color edits)

Lentils, page 108 - Justinc
https://commons.wikimedia.org/wiki/File:3_types_of_lentil.jpg (Cropped & color edits)

Parsnips, page 112, Swiss Chard page 99 - Robert
Melissa's Produce, www.melissas.com
(Cropped & color edits)

Rampion, page 115 - Eden, Janine and Jim
www.flickr.com/photos/10485077@N06/47985172326
(Cropped & color edits)

Sea kale, page 116 - Nick Smith
https://commons.wikimedia.org/wiki/File:Sea_Kale_growing_on_the_beach_-_geograph.org.uk_-_995554.jpg
(Cropped & color edits)

Skirret, page 117 - Mandy Barber
www.incrediblevegetables.co.uk
(Cropped & color edits)

Spearmint leaves, page 118, 110 - Forest and Kim Starr
https://commons.wikimedia.org/wiki/File:Starr-080607-7278-Mentha_spicata-leaves-Greenhouse_behind_galley_Sand_Island-Midway_Atoll_(38081384534).jpg
(Cropped & color edits)

Bulgur, page 96 - Johann Jaritz
https://commons.wikimedia.org/wiki/File:Bulgur_lose_26022015_8675.jpg
(Cropped & color edits)

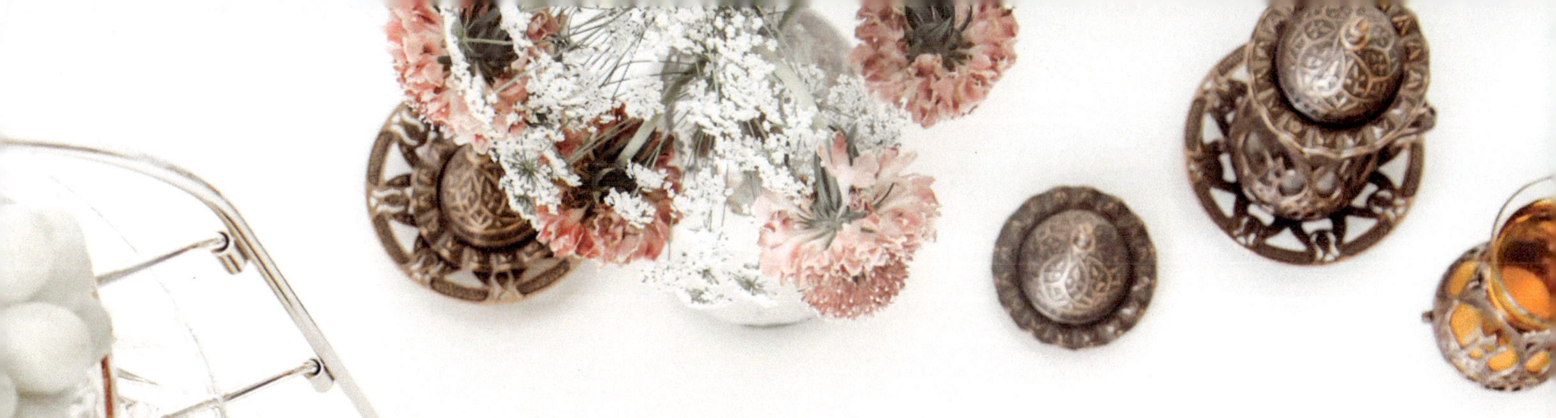

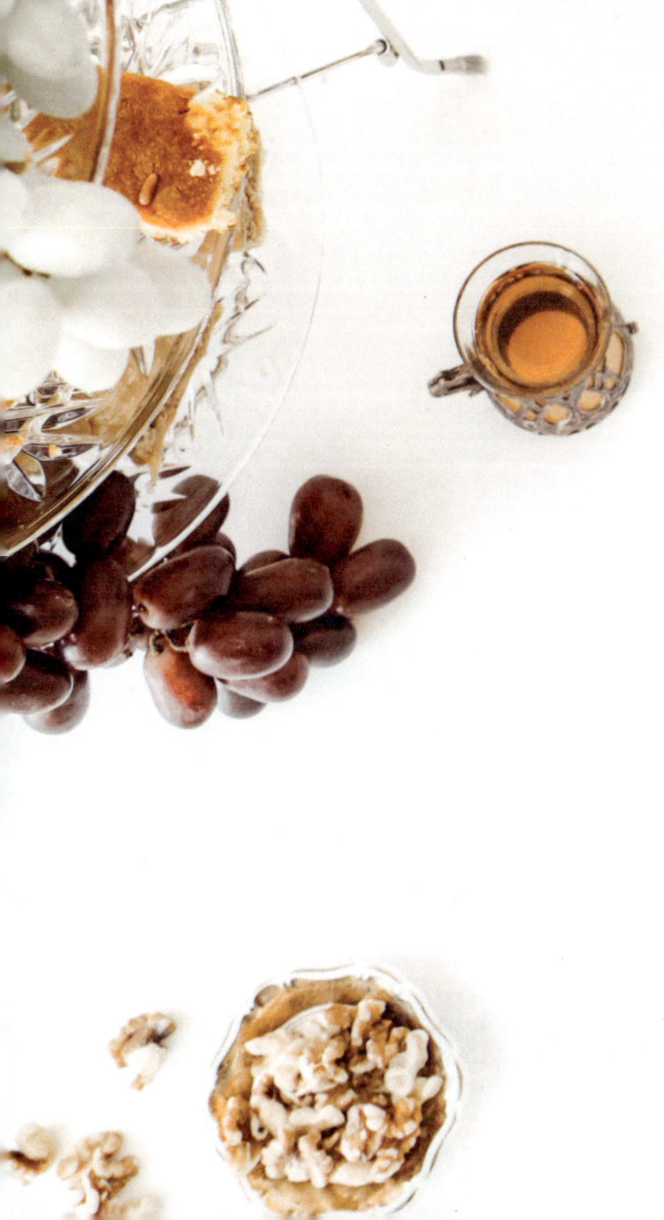

Nour invites you to share her personal journey to veganism.

From her childhood in Lebanon, learning at her grandmother's side, to her decision to become a vegan and move to America, Nour shares her story, favorite recipes, and why she is passionate about her convictions. If you are exploring veganism or feel the need for inspiration, *Vegan with Nour* is your first step into a wider world.

$24.99
ISBN 978-1-7347619-0-0
52499>
9 781734 761900

Made in United States
Cleveland, OH
29 September 2025

20899433R00081